A Dose of Madness!

Prednisone—Cure or Curse?

Dear Pastor Joe,
I really enjoyed your teaching on miracles.
This is my story that is filled with miracles, from God!
Sincerely,
Sheree May

Sheree May

ISBN 979-8-88832-578-0 (paperback)
ISBN 979-8-88832-579-7 (digital)

Copyright © 2023 by Sheree May

All rights reserved. No part of this publication may be reproduced, distributed, or transmitted in any form or by any means, including photocopying, recording, or other electronic or mechanical methods without the prior written permission of the publisher. For permission requests, solicit the publisher via the address below.

Christian Faith Publishing
832 Park Avenue
Meadville, PA 16335
www.christianfaithpublishing.com

Printed in the United States of America

CONTENTS

Foreword v
Acknowledgments vii
Chapter 1: David's Hometown 1
Chapter 2: Sheree's Hometown 12
Chapter 3: Swept Off My Feet 17
Chapter 4: Knocked Off My Feet! 27
Chapter 5: Mercy for the Dead 38
Chapter 6: My Second Wind 42
Chapter 7: A Bitter Pill to Swallow 54
Chapter 8: On My Feet Again 68
Chapter 9: The Promise 72
Chapter 10: When One Door Closes 78
Appendix A: Sheree's Journal Entries 83
Appendix B: Poems by David May (1978) 100
Appendix C: Poem by Robert Frost 110

FOREWORD

The original title my sister had chosen for this book was "King of My Castle." She had intended for it to be a tribute to her late husband. After reviewing the manuscript for her, however, I suggested a new title. While my brother-in-law was very supportive during my sister's illness, that is not what jumped out at me as I was reading.

To me, this book is about a couple working together with true grit and determination to survive a life-threatening illness in spite of a seriously flawed medical system. As a certified health coach, I was astonished to learn that no one had ever bothered to ask my sister about her nutrition!

In the pages that follow, get ready to cry, laugh, and be disappointed, angry, and downright amazed as you journey with my sister in the fight for her life. My hope is that you will get to know and appreciate my sister and brother-in-law for the struggle they went through as much as I do.

Debra Williams, IIN CHC

ACKNOWLEDGMENTS

My sincere appreciation and gratitude to the following.

My Lord and Savior Jesus Christ, who picked me up and carried me when things got so bad. I am blessed to have this opportunity to showcase God's amazing grace in my life!

Debra Williams, my supportive sister, who is my mentor and best friend. Your contribution to the content in this book is priceless. Again, you have went above and beyond!

My loving daughter, Christie Eve Dale, for taking the time to read my manuscript and provide valuable input. I love you so much!

David's daughter Leslie May, for your visits to St. Louis and for sending zucchini bread in the mail during the holidays; both always seemed to lift our spirits during the lowest point in our lives.

My mother, Helen Kennebrew, who left her job at the nursing home to care for me. Your sponge baths were cleansing in so many ways!

Dr. Erin Bakanas of Internal Medicine at St. Louis University Hospital. You saw me as a whole person and took into consideration my emotional, psychological, and physical well-being from the first day I came into your examining room. I am so grateful for the care you provided me!

Lastly, my late husband, David May, who I know is watching over me. Without your love, this book would not have existed. I wrote this book so your grandchildren Aicha and Ryan Chibani can get to know the kind of man you were during your latter years!

CHAPTER 1

David's Hometown

Perryville, my husband's birth city, was named for Commodore Oliver Hazard Perry, a naval hero of the War of 1812. In 1821, Perryville was selected as the county seat. Until the year 1824, the population of the county consisted chiefly of Shawnee and Delaware Indians. Once the land in Perry became known for its fertility, Germans and French immigrated there. It is said that Perryville had the good fortune to be settled by a class of people remarkable for their intelligence, honesty, and uprightness. It was also claimed that religion and education were more honored there than any other place on earth.

The Catholic population of Perryville needed a permanent resident priest and offered 640 acres of land to Bishop Louis William Valentine DuBourg in exchange for the regular services of a priest and a school for the children.

It is written that the founding of St. Mary's of the Barrens in Perryville, Missouri, predates the founding of the State of Missouri by two years. It was the first seminary west of the Mississippi River. The Roman Catholic church and seminary was founded by the Vincentians, a member of the Roman Catholic Congregation of the Mission founded by St. Vincent de Paul in Paris, France, in 1625 and devoted to missions and seminaries. St. Mary's of the Barrens seminary was established in October 1818.

The seminary at Perryville was the official seminary of the entire St. Louis diocese until 1842, when the diocesan seminary was moved to St. Louis. Thereafter, St. Mary's was reserved only for training Vincentian seminarians.

In 1880, Charles A. Weber was elected as first mayor of Perryville. With the building of the Chester, Perryville and St. Genevieve Railway, prosperity came. Largely because of its role as the seat of county government and because of its central location, Perryville began to develop as the major commercial and service center in Perry County. The population increased from 897 in 1890 to 1,275 in 1900.

The traditional heart of Perryville was the courthouse square. The centerpiece of the square was the Perry County Courthouse. In 1913, the first power plant was built to provide Perryville with electric lights. The chamber of commerce was formed in 1923 and launched one of the first economic development efforts in the nation. After raising $100,000 and building one of the first industrial spec buildings, the International Shoe Company was persuaded to expand their operations by opening a Perryville plant. The population boomed again, more than doubling from 1,763 in 1920 to 3,907 in 1940.

The May family was a part of that population. David's mother, Marie May, worked at the shoe plant. She was known for her efficiency and work ethic. It was said that the other employees couldn't keep up with her fast pace on the assembly line.

In 1978, David wrote about the town he grew up in and titled it "A Lot of Us Came from One":

> The town was small by all standards. Except by those who lived there. We've all seen them somewhere. A lot of us came from one. Those who have and those who haven't all made the classic joke, "Don't blink as you drive by, or you'll miss it."
> Dominating the town square is the red of the brick courthouse surrounded by trees, shade, grass, and green benches for the old men to sit and watch the town grow old. Resting there for generations never to witness anything new. The only change in all those years are two electric traffic lights at opposite ends of the square.

The show's humble marquee hangs on the westside. Two soda fountains enjoyed on the north. To the south, hardware is the main business. Bank and so-called general store are somewhere in between; grocery around the corner. The east side, well, it houses the five saloons inside.

Those in town worked at making shoes; the farmers nested around the edges.

Families of twelve were not uncommon. Seemed like relatives were everywhere. At family reunions, you'd swear you were a cousin to everyone in town.

Fish fries were popular. Big ones for church affairs; little ones for neighbors. Catfish was the favorite, but they had a lot of bones. On St. Blaise Day, the priest would bless every throat, which made me think of catfish and all those bones on St. Blaise Day.

It's a good town to grow up in; plenty of room and plenty of time to go frog gigging along the creeks or catch pigeons in old barns at night with gunny sacks and flashlights. Kids can drive a hard bargain for a matched pair of all whites. Then there was flashlight tag at night with the city limits as boundary lines.

There were two policemen. One was old Charlie Alkameyer. He was nice and friendly. I met him at the school cross. The other one I didn't know much about. Only two things stood out about him. Wrecking his police car into a tree, he claimed the tree moved. Another was he shot his car and put three bullet holes in the hood. I didn't think too much of him.

There were plenty of chores too with our own truck patch out back. Mom was smart enough to buy three ironing boards, each a different size to match the height of her three sons.

She grew up in a place called Dry Bone. One didn't have to see to know what it was like. The name told it all. What could be worse than a farmer calling his own land "Dry Bone"? It was a hard life. That place produced hard people. Mother was the kindliest, the gentlest of them all. She was much chided about her thriftiness. A place called Dry Bone was responsible.

Mother was always canning something or making jelly from the grapes she picked at St. Mary's vineyard for a dollar a bushel. And woe to the boy who let the jelly boil over while sitting on a stool next to the stove reading a comic book. It was never too hard to con my grandma into shaking the big gallon of cream with the hope that, by nightfall, it would shake into a ball of butter. I was lucky enough to have a grandma living with me.

Snapping beans and hulling peas while sitting in the white rocker helped pass the lazy summer days. It did have its drawbacks though. My thumb became so tender and sore. I could hardly bear to touch it, especially with my boyish bad habit of biting my fingernails. Chewed nails was very embarrassing when I served the six o'clock Mass, and the priest, immaculate in his white vestments, looked down at my hands as I passed the water and wine cruets.

Church was a big part of my life. Mass every morning before school. The church is St. Boniface, smaller than the town deserved. Farther out, amid old trees, stood a larger edifice ringed by apple orchards, dairy barns, stretching vineyards, and grazing Black Angus. For all, only one name serves St. Mary's of the Barrens.

I rolled a lot of beads between my fingers. I said a lot of beads on my knees and practiced those Latin lines in order to serve Mass. It was hard. But oh, I was so proud reciting them out loud. Some kids drank the altar wine, but some were too scared.

It was quiet in Perryville, except on Sundays. It was just a little quieter.

Christmas was a big time. It seems like the flakes were always feet deep when only a kid. Outside I'd go; snowballs to make. The long red sled with kids piled high, downhill it slid. My friends would help build forts of snow; pack them in ice so they would keep. Sides were taken, and raids were planned; theirs to attack, ours to defend. The play went on and on. My feet frozen and my hands numb. The fall of night and Mother's call forced us inside, where I was tucked in tight.

Morning brought the sun. The adults were glad, but us kids were sad. Those proud fortresses were now a memory. Their walls packed in ice laid down in the warmth. Time for a new fun.

If somehow I forgot, I knew it was Christmas from the peanut brittle stacked high on the cut glass plate. I ate more than I ought; gone till next year this date.

Santa came Christmas Eve. And even though it was Uncle Lonnie dressed in a red suit with a big pillow, I didn't care pretending to believe.

All went to midnight Mass, so glad to be singing with all those in my class. Most got there early to tell the others what had been hiding for them under the tree.

A few of the children were chosen the next day to sing inside the courthouse. Their voices, mingling with the season's air, warmed those who were half frozen all around the square.

Football was the town sport. Having a large truck patch in back and a father who plowed it for the fall. Six inches of soft dirt made for a soft landing.

Mother didn't like it much. Oh, she complained a lot about the dust and that sort of thing. But everyone knew there must have been a reason why she let it continue. Under all the complaints, her heart was touched watching her sons play ball.

At the Brewers' house, lights were strung in rows over the backyard. Even night didn't stop the football. The ground was marked for boundaries and yard lines. Two large stones were put in place to mark the goal lines. One of my friends painted "Gold" on each of the stones. Mrs. Brewer tried in vain to convince him it should be spelled "Goal." He would have none of it. After all, she was so old, and he was so wise.

If tired of football, softball and swimming were our summer sports. Every town had its swimming hole. This one was called Saline Creek. It was several miles west of town.

Saline Creek was green with patches of white foam that sometimes floated by. But broader and deeper was my favorite swimming spot. A brown sandy shore on the far side; on the near side was a sloping gray boulder split down the middle five foot wide. That's why they called it Split-Rock Creek. Some teased about a yellow streak if too afraid to make that leap. There was a red blotch near the split. Story goes a boy tried to jump but slipped, and his chin caught the rock. Sounded like the kind of gory tale kids at the swimming hole liked to tell.

Most of the summer I would spend on my front porch. I would sit in the white rocker on the big red porch and rock and rock and rock all day.

Rocking was good on rainy days, when the skies were black, the wind had its way, and rain splattered hard on the street. This was the time, of course, when all big thinking was done. Daydreams were best. I could remember them, whereas dreams at night were soon forgotten. There must have been lots of rainy days because I did a lot of rocking.

Mother began to fret about so much rocking. Especially if it wasn't a rainy day.

I was sent to the hospital. There, I was told something about polio. It was a scary thought for one not so old. I had my suspicions for my visit. The doctor had glasses and a red beard. He said nothing as he stared at me. Mother visited me at the hospital and said very little.

Doctors and parents talked in a whisper, far enough away so I couldn't hear. It turned out, I didn't have what they feared, and the rocking continued with my daydreams. I was going to be pope and president.

David spent most of his adolescent years preparing to become a Catholic priest. He graduated from St. Vincent's College ("The Cape") Preparatory Seminary of the Congregation of the Mission on May 24, 1959.

It is recorded in "The Cape" yearbook:

> The life of a seminarian includes a balanced program of activities and studies which tends to supply him with the greatest possible assistance in attaining his priestly goal. There is no small

phase or function in his seminary life which is not consistent with the vocation which he has chosen. Every detail, regulation, or activity is ordered to the seminarian's development.

The religious life of one who strives to be "another Christ" is emphasized, for the spirituality of the priest and his work is his distinguishing mark. The seminarian learns to appreciate the Sacrifice of the Mass, which he hopes to offer one day. He is instilled with a greater knowledge and understanding of the Sacraments and the Church; and, by means of daily meditation, spiritual reading, and recitation of the Rosary, he brings himself to a fuller recognition of his supernatural life and spiritual needs.

The education of the seminarian is also obviously important. His studies correspond with the studies of the outside schools, with more emphasis placed on certain subjects necessary to his vocation. History, mathematics, social studies, and English are indispensable to any man. The priest, therefore, a teacher of men, must thoroughly equip himself with such knowledge in order to perform the duties of his call in life. Latin, being the official tongue of the Church, is necessarily stressed, and its importance committed to the applicants to the Priesthood.

Recreation has always been recognized as being as important to the seminarian's makeup as his other activities. A man must be healthy if he wishes to enter into labor for Christ. And this is the aim of the seminary—to fit a boy physically and mentally for the Priesthood. Plentiful facilities for all sports and games, ranging from baseball, basketball, and football to handball, swimming, and tennis, supply the students with the needed recreation. But aside from recreational purposes, it is also believed that such sports develop in the seminarian a sense of sportsmanship and good feeling, so necessary in his later work.

Extracurricular activities give the student a chance to develop certain talents which he may possess. The various clubs (camera, dramatic, and glee) are designed for the special interests of the students in these fields. If a student enjoys group and choral singing, he may be a member of the Glee Club. For those who are interested in photography, the Camera Club provides ample instructions and the facilities necessary to develop their photographic skills. Varied types of plays are regularly presented by the Dramatics Club, whose members prefer acting to music and photography.

The Clients of Mary and Joseph has been a prominent organization at Cape ever since its foundation over fifty years ago, it has been firmly established as an extracurricular activity in which all the students participate. The primary purpose of the meetings is to give each student an opportunity to make any suggestion which, in his opinion, will be of advantage to the student body. If these suggestions, after being thoroughly discussed, are still judged profitable to the student body, each member has the duty to carry them out to the best of his ability. Thus, by their very nature, the meetings tend to develop a high degree of initiative, responsibility, and character in all the clients. The debating, discussion, and exchange of ideas serves to develop the ability in the students to "think on their feet," to express themselves clearly, and to gain poise in public speaking, qualities which will play a great part in their later lives when called upon to deliver sermons or to speak extemporaneously before some group.

As a rule, Client meetings are held every Tuesday night. The meetings start with prayers, followed by the singing of the Ave Maria, then, after the roll call, the minutes of the last meeting are read. Hereupon an appointed student gives a news report, and another student a sports report. The president then turns the floor to questions of general welfare. It is at this point that the students offer their ideas on ways and means to improve themselves or how they may better some facet of life here at Cape. After all business has been taken care of, a motion for adjournment is raised and seconded. The meeting is closed with prayers for our benefactors and our foreign missions. All sessions are conducted according to parliamentary procedures. In such organized meetings, much more can be accomplished than in any other way.

All in all, these clubs and organizations add the needed variety to fill out the seminary's round of activities.

Apart from the scheduled curricular, such as clubs and sports, the student body of the seminary also looks forward to Mardi Gras and its accompanying floats submitted by each class, the annual bazaar with its games and prizes; the trip to Perryville; and all the other added treats, such as Halloween, the Christmas and the Easter banquets, and the oratorical contests. A seminarian knows no such thing as a dull moment!

During his four years in the minor seminary, the seminarian is given various tasks and jobs to perform, which not only add to the upkeep and appearance of the seminary building and grounds, but which also contribute to the formation of character. Responsibility, one of the most important traits of a priest, is thus singularized and impressed upon the seminarian in the earliest stages of his character development. It is firmly believed that, by accepting the burden and responsibility of small tasks, the priest-to-be may be experienced and prepared to shoulder the *heavier duties of his later life.*

There is not a single function of the entire priestly studies of the seminarian which has not been designed with a definite and important purpose in mind. The seminary life is a happy life. It is a complete and well-fitted life from its first years to its last. Whether a man completes the studies or not, the seminary will have *left its mark and character upon him, and through him, upon the world!*

David grew up preparing to become a priest. However, after six-plus years of seminary life, he left for the big city. It was there that his life took a 180-degree turn. He met and married a beautiful lady named Barbara and had a family. He studied to become a lawyer; they later divorced.

David then moved to Florida, where he took over a White Wall business while living with a lady named Marilyn. That relationship ended, and shortly afterward, David moved back to St. Louis to be near his brother, Donald. The two of them worked in sales.

After two marriages and one long-term relationship, David met me. We were the unlikely pair, the boy from Perryville, Missouri, and the girl from East St. Louis, Illinois. David was seventeen years older than me chronologically. Intellectually, we were on the same level.

CHAPTER 2

Sheree's Hometown

History reveals that in the early 1870s, Mayor John Bowman had envisioned a new stockyard operation in East St. Louis. It would rival the famous Union Stock Yards in Chicago and make the stockyards in nearby St. Louis minor by comparison. He approached a group of wealthy investors about establishing it.

Construction began on May 30, 1871. It is said that $1.5 million was spent to construct the complex. It included 100 acres of animal pens, 60 acres for sheds, and the Allerton House (later known as the National Hotel), where Theodore Roosevelt once stayed. It was the finest hotel in the area.

National City was a town incorporated in 1907 to counter the increasing intervention of government into the company's affairs. It was a company town owned by the National Stockyards. The town consisted of two streets a block long, with about forty houses, a building that served as a church and school, a police/fire station, and a store. The village had a population of approximately 300, all of whom were employees of the stockyards. Everything in town was under the direct control of the company, from the mayor (hand-picked by the company) to the tax assessments. This control allowed the company to efficiently run its own affairs with minimal outside governmental interference such as taxation and regulation. National City was the first industrial suburb outside East St. Louis.

The stockyards were built to accommodate 15,000 head of cattle; 10,000 sheep; and 20,000 hogs. By 1938, 60 percent of the livestock shipped to National City came by trucks instead of by trains; and by 1952, that number grew to 99 percent of hogs and 84 percent of all other animals.

My grandparents lived a few blocks from the National Stockyards in a place called Goose Hill. My grandmother Mary cleaned offices at the St. Louis National Stockyards. My grandfather Willie worked in "hog kill" at Hunter Packing Company, which was located across the street from his home.

My mother, Helen, was the seventh child of ten girls. I was nine years old when my mom divorced her first husband and moved back to Goose Hill. I quickly grew immune to the stench of hogs being transported into town on 18-wheelers. The trucks drove through town day and night. I would wake up and go to bed to the sound of squealing hogs being driven to Hunter's to be slaughtered.

Life on Goose Hill, an area of East St. Louis, Illinois, moved by the sound of the whistle from the smokestack that sat on the rooftop of the Hunter Packing Company. The whistle blew for the first shift, at lunchtime, and when it was time to go home.

It was a good town to grow up in. The town was about one mile long and one mile wide. Everyone knew everyone, it seems. There were barbecues every holiday. Everyone in town was always welcomed. Families of ten or more were not uncommon. It seemed like everyone was related on Goose Hill. There was one park in town near Garfield Elementary School, the only elementary school in town for preschool to third grade. Everyone would gather at the park on holidays for barbecue ribs.

I could always tell when it was Sunday on Goose Hill; no 18-wheelers came to town. It had two Baptist churches. My sister and I were baptized at Southern Mission Baptist Church by Reverend Gee. Our family spent the first part of the day in church, where most of us sung in the choir. Then we had dinner at Grandma's, which was my favorite thing to do. My grandmother was known for her sweet tooth, and her kitchen always smelled of baked cakes or cobblers.

There were also block parties on Goose Hill. The town always knew how to let off steam after working all week long in a meatpacking plant. People traveled from all over East St. Louis and beyond to work at Hunter's.

Goose Hill was not only surrounded by one of the largest stockyards and several meat-processing plants, but the town was also surrounded by railroad tracks. I remember spending most of my childhood sitting in the back seat of Uncle Jack's car, watching the trains pass by. I always imagined the many places I could go if I just climbed onboard. I wondered how many towns like mine the trains went through. I pictured the life of a hobo to be filled with adventure, unlike life on Goose Hill, which was filled with hard hats, goggles, and bloody white frocks draped around tired bodies.

My mom worked at the Hunter Packing Company. She was a "pork boner." She started at $12 per hour, which was considered a lot of money in the '60s. My mom always came home from work exhausted. She would pass out in her bed until it was time to go back to work. On weekends, she would sleep in on Saturdays and go to church on Sunday. My mom told us that she didn't want that sort of life for her children. She stressed to us how important a good education was. As a result, both of her daughters went to college. Her youngest (my sister, Debra) graduated from Northwestern University in Evanston, Illinois, with a bachelor's in computer science. Her oldest (that's me) received a master's in mass communication from Southern Illinois University in Edwardsville, Illinois.

I was in my second year of graduate school and still unsure of my career path. I had recently been hired as news editor of our campus newspaper. I had an appointment to interview the mayor of East St. Louis. I was nervous about the interview, which was scheduled to take place tomorrow. I was going to interview the person who was blamed for the city's huge debt.

On July 1989, I was walking to the bus stop on my way to class when the smells of spoiled fish and sour milk overwhelmed me. I passed spilled-over trashcans and stepped over soiled diapers strewn along the sidewalks by alley cats and stray dogs. I covered my nose with my hand as I clawed my way through filth and garbage to reach my destination.

Here is an article in the *Chicago Tribune* by J. A. Lobbia published on April 5, 1989:

> EAST ST. LOUIS—Just when it looked like the only way things in East St. Louis could go was up, the city took another slide backward last week.
>
> Mayor Carl Officer failed to show up Friday for a hearing on the city's decrepit sewer system and faces contempt-of-court charges at a hearing scheduled for April 14 by St. Clair County judge Sheila O'Brien, who said she was "disgusted" with Officer's behavior.
>
> In February, O'Brien had ordered the city to make repairs in the sewer system after it began returning raw sewage into schools and homes.
>
> The deteriorated system is only one of the myriad serious problems that continue to plague East St. Louis's 55,000 people. Among others:
>
> —Late last month, Officer asked the unions representing the city's 238 workers to take a 50 percent pay cut. As it is, workers have not been paid for about a month and have lost their health benefits because the city no longer can afford them, said city personnel director Kelvin Ellis.
>
> —Last Thursday, the school board announced it was sending layoff notices to about half of the district's 1,800 employees and was planning to actually lay off between 300 and 500, including teachers, because of financial difficulties.
>
> The city has not picked up trash for more than a year; it can't pay the garbage hauler it hired.
>
> City debt is about $50 million.

Every news article on Mayor Carl Officer read similar. I didn't look forward to adding more fuel to the fire. I wanted to do something to lift my city, not keep it down with more negative publicity. The interview was not successful. No matter how I tried to make the mayor seem like he wanted what was best for the city, I had no hard evidence to support it. I couldn't see myself as an effective reporter.

I cried that I had spent six years in college and still had no clear vision of where I was headed in life. I was a divorced mother of a teenager. My mom had been caring for my daughter while I tried to better my life after a bad marriage. I wanted to do something meaningful with my life. I just didn't know what.

I grew up listening to fairy tales. I grew up waiting to be rescued by a prince. Instead, I was in an unfaithful marriage that left me a single parent who was so busy trying to better myself that I missed raising my daughter.

I enrolled in Central Baptist Seminary (located in Kansas) the following summer after I received my master's. It was through a lot of praying for guidance that led me there. My boyfriend at the time told me, if I left, don't bother returning. Our five-year relationship ended when I told him I was going into the seminary.

Though I excelled in my studies at the seminary, I decided to go back home the following fall. I felt I had to go back and repair my damaged relationship with my teenage daughter. She had gotten out of control. It was time for me to own up to my responsibilities. The only way I could do that was find a full-time job.

I had been in school for such a long time. My dream job was to write for major print media, like a popular magazine such as *Good Housekeeping* or a big city newspaper like the *St. Louis Post-Dispatch*! I had the education but not the experience. After unsuccessful attempts at applying at local newspapers and other media, I became self-employed. I started working at the only job I could get at the time, and there I met David May.

CHAPTER 3

Swept Off My Feet

On October 6, 1991, David and I married.

Anyone who would see us at first glance would not consider us a couple. David was a fifty-year-old penny-pinching, hot-tempered Caucasian extrovert who smoked two packs of cigarettes a day and loved to voice his political views to anyone who listened.

I, on the other hand, was a thirty-three-year-old African American introvert who didn't smoke, cared what everyone thought of me, and always tried to buy my friends.

David and I met in a bar. He captured my attention because he was the only one who wasn't drunk. He was sipping on a club soda. I walked up to him and asked if he was drinking club soda because he was a recovering alcoholic. He said no. He told me that he had just lost 170 lb., and he didn't want to start adding the pounds back by drinking alcohol. I was impressed by the amount of weight he said he had lost. I listened attentively as he told me how he did it.

During our first date, I learned that David had spent most of his childhood (including adolescence) in a seminary. The conversation we had was unlike any I'd had on previous dates. David was smart. We were both college graduates and had attended seminaries. He enjoyed photography. I enjoyed dancing. I told him that I wanted to spend my younger years traveling the world as a famous dancer. And then in my forties, I wanted to come back to St. Louis and work at the *St. Louis Post-Dispatch*. I didn't know why, but I always wanted to work there in advertising.

David said that when he was a young boy, he wanted to be both pope and president. I truly believed he was smart enough to pull it off. The only thing that would prevent that from happening was his lifestyle. He had left the seminary, been married twice, and his conversation was full of obscenity and profanity. Yet the more I spent time with David, the more I got to see his passion and his sense of humor, which I fell in love with. He made me smile and laugh a lot. He could always comfort me when I was at my worst, especially when he would sing the Gregorian chant he learned during his life in the seminary. I never understood the words because the words were in Latin. Yet I loved to hear him sing to me in Latin. It always made me smile.

David introduced me to a new world. He got me involved in politics. He took me on my first camping trip. He also took me on my first trip to Vegas, which I knew was going to be very special.

David kept telling me about the chapels in Vegas. He said he couldn't wait to take me to see them. I took that as a sign that he was going to ask me to marry him. I felt he was going to pop the question in Vegas. I was never into big weddings. I wanted something small and intimate.

We had only been dating a few months. I'd known my first husband since childhood, and that marriage didn't last a year. I knew I wanted to be David's wife only a month after we met. My first impression of him was a good one. I was in love with his knowledge of history and of the Catholic religion. I admired how he never cared what people thought. He would be a loyal and loving husband. I would be his third wife. He would be my second husband. We both had learned a lot from our previous marriages.

The minute the plane landed in Vegas, I was bombarded with lights and the *cha-ching* of slot machines! I had never seen so many blinking, flashing lights. It was like Christmas in paradise. I froze like a deer in headlights. I just stood in place because there was so much to look at that I didn't know which way to turn. I felt as if I had landed on another planet. There were people everywhere from everywhere. They spoke all kinds of different languages.

David and I checked into our hotel. He then took me to dinner at the buffet. There was so much food to choose from. It was the first time I tried prime rib. It was the best food I had ever tasted. We walked on the strip after we ate. We went inside Caesars Palace, where David showed me how to play blackjack. I loved the decor inside Caesars. It was like stepping into the Roman Empire. There was a twenty-foot statue of Augustus Caesar at the entrance. The staff wore Greco-Roman wigs and Roman costumes. It was an atmosphere I enjoyed for hours.

The following day, after a hearty breakfast, David and I visited the chapels. They were nothing like what I expected. They weren't nearly as glamorous on the inside like the casinos. I was underwhelmed. The chapels were small and quaint. We had toured several, but I couldn't pick out one to be married in. I felt them to be very cold and impersonal. The vibe I got when I walked into Caesar's was not the vibe I got when I walked into the chapels.

After we toured the last chapel, David and I went shopping. He took me inside a jewelry store. We looked around. He asked me if anything caught my eye. I tried on rings. I was so excited, I could hardly hold it in. I didn't want to spoil the surprise for David. I didn't know what he had planned for the proposal.

We left the jewelry store and headed to lunch. As we were walking, David said he had left something back at the store. He asked me to sit on the bench nearby until he returned. I knew what he was up to. He was going to purchase one of the rings I had tried on. I was smiling inside at the thought of going back home a married woman. I was going to make David one happy man!

David returned and we proceeded to lunch. While eating lunch, I was trying to imagine what he had planned for that evening. Our plane would leave for home tomorrow evening. I knew he would propose during or after dinner that day, and we would head to the chapel that night. I was going to put on my elegant black leather minidress with my six-inch heels. I was beginning to feel like Cinderella.

I was eighteen years old when I married my first husband. I have one daughter from that marriage. I am now in my early thirties. Soon I wouldn't be able to have children. It was time to settle down in case I wanted to have more children. David and I had not talked about having children. He had two daughters from his first marriage. Together, we had three girls. He probably would like to have a son.

After dinner that evening, I was on the edge of my seat when David reached into his pocket. He pulled out a small box and handed it to me. I was a little taken aback when he didn't get on one knee. I thought how lazy of him not to adhere to the tradition. I opened the box, knowing that he was getting ready to ask me to marry him. Suddenly, my whole expression went from happy to shock. I closed then opened my eyes again to make sure I was seeing what I was seeing. I wasn't staring down at one of the rings I had tried on. I was staring down at a blue sewing thimble.

I looked up at David and asked if this was some sort of prank. He said it was the only thing he could afford in the jewelry store. I told him I didn't sew, nor did I want to learn to sew. He said he bought it as a memento of our first time in Vegas together. I didn't know if I should put it back in the box or throw it at him. I wasn't one to make a scene, so I just put it away as I held back the tears.

I didn't speak much that evening. I guess I was still in shock. I just wanted to go home and try to forget everything that had just happened. David noticed that my whole demeanor had changed. He asked me what was wrong. I couldn't believe he couldn't see what was wrong. I couldn't talk to him about it. I was too emotional. I just said that nothing was wrong and became silent the rest of the evening.

I didn't say much to David for days after we returned home. When I finally brought up the subject, David said that he cared about our relationship too much to demean it by getting married at a chapel in Vegas. He also wanted to share such a special event with some of our closest family and friends. He made me see how inconsiderate I would have been to marry him in Vegas without my mother and daughter present. After all, it was only a few months later that we started planning our wedding. The planning had been just as special as the actual event. I will never forget the night he proposed.

David took me on a carriage ride near the St. Louis Gateway Arch after having a steak dinner at the famous Dierdorf & Hart's

Steakhouse. He got on one knee inside the carriage, which was parked along the riverfront. It was a perfect night! David proposed to me underneath a sky full of stars. I wouldn't have wanted it any other way.

David and I spent a lot of time planning our wedding and honeymoon while walking on the six-mile bike path in Forest Park. That trail was very special because it's where David lost his 170 lb. only a year ago. He said that he would do two laps around that trail at one time. I couldn't even do a half lap. He would have to go and get the car halfway through the trail. I told him I didn't know how he was able to walk around that complete trail twice.

He was a chain-smoker. He would always have a lit Winston pressed between his lips while walking on the bike path. Joggers would pass us and tell David that smoking was bad for his health. He would respond by telling them that it was his health, not theirs, and to mind their own business. People on the trail would also tell him to put out his cigarette because he was in a no-smoking zone. He would tell them to go take a hike.

I was always embarrassed by David's behavior. He would see the disappointment on my face and start doing little silly things like skipping down the path to find a daffodil to pick and put in my hair. I would then smile at him and shake my head.

We spent a lot of time walking in Forest Park. David and I had so much to discuss during our walks. We decided on a small and inexpensive wedding followed by a long and extravagant honeymoon. Neither of us were much for big social events.

Our wedding took place on October 6, 1991, in our two-bedroom condominium that overlooked the St. Louis skyline including the Gateway Arch. There were a dozen roses and a few guests from our immediate family. I walked down the staircase and into the family room to the song "Edelweiss" from the *Sound of Music*. I was in a white sleeveless sundress and holding a red rose. David was standing in front of the female minister whom we'd found on the internet.

I will always remember what she said to me after the ceremony. The minister walked up to me, looked me straight in the eyes, and said that she could tell that my words came from a great spirit. Could she have been referring to the wedding vows I wrote to my husband?

> David,
> You are my king, I am your queen
> And God is our "e ver y thing!"
>
> I was once lost, and you were alone.
> Your place and my place were no place we wanted to call home.
> Apart we hummed different tunes. Your Latin chant pushed away my blues.
> Your time and my time meant there was no time to lose.
>
> You are my king, I am your queen
> And faith is our "e ver y thing!"
>
> Our two religions will intertwine.
> Together we will become one, as our two faiths combine.
> Together we will sow obedience and will reap humility.
> Together we will sow grace and reap dignity!
>
> You are my king, I am your queen
> And grace is our "e ver y thing!"
>
> Your words have truth, and my words have heart
> Together they work miracles and chaos when apart
> Our differences were obvious, but together they made us strong
> And our life will inspire an "a ma a zing" song!
>
> You are my king, I am your queen
> And God is always "eve ry thing!"

I didn't know what to make of the minister's comment, so I took it as a compliment.

David and I started our honeymoon right after the reception dinner. We packed up our car and headed to Yosemite National Park that evening. We were in the car for hours upon hours. We started taking turns driving every hour just to keep from dozing. We drove in and out of darkness. After a day and a half, we pulled into a little town tucked away in the foothills of the Colorado Rockies. The town was called Nederland. We checked into the only hotel in town and then took a stroll into the heart of town, where we found a great Italian restaurant.

Though we noticed that the sun had dropped behind the mountains after dinner, I wanted to take a leisurely stroll before resting for the night. We didn't walk very far before we were enveloped in total darkness. I couldn't see David or my hand in front of me. There were no streetlights, and the moon was nowhere in sight. I told my husband this had been a bad idea. We turned around quickly and headed back the way we came. I was glad the town was very small. We fumbled our way back to the hotel.

The following morning, we got back on the road. On our way out of town, we passed a family of deer taking a sip from a nearby creek just at the edge of town.

We drove through Rocky Mountain National Park. The views were astounding. Our next destination was Lake Tahoe, Nevada. David and I were going to spend a couple of days there before heading to our final destination.

The weather seemed to be in our favor. The days were sunny and nice, and the nights were quiet and clear. After another two days of highway driving, we arrived at Lake Tahoe on a moonlit night.

We drove around a calm, glistening body of water that stretched beneath a sky full of stars. The stars were dancing on top of the lake. The twinkling scene brought a certain warmth on a chilly night in October. My husband and I spent a very relaxing night in a room at the Holiday Inn.

Lake Tahoe had such a calming effect on me. David and I went horseback riding on trails that overlooked the lake. The next day, we took to the mountains on foot. We went hiking on trails with steep slopes and narrow dirt paths. David always gave me the heavy backpack while he only carried his water canteen. His excuse was that I was much younger and in better shape. He'd then reach into his top pocket for his pack of Winston cigarettes and light one before continuing on the trail.

There were breathtaking views all around us. We would stop and take in the scenery. My husband would take the camera out of our backpack and snap away. He always liked me to be in the pictures. He was a perfectionist and would have me posing for what seemed like forever before he took the shot. Sometimes I felt like an overworked, unpaid model!

Our next adventure during our stay in Lake Tahoe took us to a small stretch of the famous Pacific Crest Trail. We went into the thick of the forest in search of a place called Sunset Meadows. The path took us miles away from any hint of civilization. I felt we were lost at times. David and I were good at wandering off the trail by mistake.

After a couple of stops during our four-mile hike through woods, brush, and thickets, we came to a wide sunny opening. My jaw dropped immediately at the sight of it. Sunset Meadows looked like a neglected wheat field. The yellow stalks had grown wild, thus hiding the meandering stream that ran through the meadow. However, it wasn't a total waste once I saw the meadow come to life. A chipmunk made its way through the tall stalks to sunbathe in the openness. A multicolored butterfly sat upon one of the tall stalks, flapping its wings in the sunlight. I listened to a woodpecker busy at work on a nearby tree. I could always see the beauty in everything.

We spent a few days in Lake Tahoe, and then we were back on the road again. We were now heading to our final destination: Yosemite National Park. The road twisted through and around the mountains. A winding stream followed us to the north entrance of Yosemite. I became worried when we passed a sign that read "Beware of Bears."

The sun started to set, and I grew anxious to get to our destination. My husband had booked a suite and brought champagne for us to make a toast. An hour later, it was pitch-dark, and our car started making strange squeaking sounds. I became frantic at the thought of getting stuck in a forest full of bears. The farther we drove, the louder the car squealed.

I asked David what was wrong with our car. He said that it sounded like the brakes were going out. I started to cry. I accused him of ruining our brakes because he didn't know how to drive in the mountains. I was angry because I didn't want to pull up to the hotel with our car sounding that way. We would wake up all the guests. People would notice us! It would be embarrassing. I didn't want people looking at us strange. I just wanted to hide under a rock.

My husband became upset at the way I was behaving. Once we arrived at the hotel, instead of being thankful, I rushed into our suite and locked myself in the bathroom. I spent the night sleeping on the bathroom floor. My husband spent the night drinking champagne by himself on the king bed.

I woke up the next morning from the sound of the door being opened. It was David coming back to tell me that he had taken the car to the shop and that our brakes were being repaired. He also said there was a shuttle stop nearby where we could catch the shuttle that would take us into Yosemite. I got dressed. We had a delicious breakfast, and then we walked to the road where we waited for the shuttle. Inside the park, we rented some bikes to tour the valley floor.

In describing Yosemite, an author named John Muir wrote the following:

> Yosemite is situated in the basin of the Merced River at an elevation of 4000 feet above sea level. It is about seven miles long, half a mile to a mile wide, and nearly a mile deep in the solid granite flank of the range. The walls are made up of rocks, mountains in size, partly separated from each other by side canyons, and they are so sheer in front, and so compactly and harmoniously arranged on a level floor, that the Valley looks like an immense hall of illuminated temples. Every rock in its wall seems to glow with life. Some lean

back in majestic repose; others, absolutely sheer for thousands of feet. Their feet among beautiful groves and meadows, their brows in the sky, a thousand flowers leaning confidently against their feet, bathed in floods of water, floods of light, while the snow and waterfalls, the winds and avalanches and clouds shine and sing about them as the years go by.

We rode our bikes first to Bridal Falls, which turned out to be just a huge dry stone where water sometimes fell from. However, the rock climbers took advantage of the dry season and attempted to climb Bridal Falls. It was a beautiful sight, a couple of tiny figures clinging against the hard surface for dear life.

David lit a Winston before we continued our bike-riding tour of Yosemite Valley. We rode by the giant Half Dome, which was a huge stone rounded at the top. We found more rock climbers making their way up the huge stone wall. There were huge carved stone walls throughout the park. The El Capitan was sheer and robust, standing straight up and down. It was a great challenge for even the best of the rock climbers.

Our next stop was at an Indian exhibition, which was about the lifestyles of the Yosemite, a tribe the park had been named after. The Indian name of the valley was Ahwahnee. It was great to touch and walk inside a tepee. I always admired how the native Indians showed a great respect for the land. The tour was enlightening.

David and I woke up the next morning, packed our bags, and headed home. The honeymoon was over. It was time for us to get back to the hustle and bustle of city life.

CHAPTER 4

Knocked Off My Feet!

Spring 1992, less than six months after our wedding, my husband and I were doing our usual stroll along the bike trail in Forest Park when he brought up the fact that we didn't have health-care insurance. He was worried that if either of us became very sick, we could lose our home. I asked him if he had been feeling ill. I wanted to know why health care had become so important to him suddenly. He said he had been watching the presidential primaries and had seen reports on how people had lost their homes and life savings when one of them became sick and didn't have any health-care coverage. David read in a report that thirty million people in the United States didn't have health care because they couldn't afford it.

My husband tried to get health-care insurance. The fact that he was a fifty-year-old chain-smoker who was slightly overweight made the premiums impossible to afford. We were both independent contractors. We would have to pay the full premiums. David purchased Blue Cross/Blue Shield health insurance for me at $76 per month. His would cost three times that amount. We decided to wait a year before he got health insurance. After all, what could go wrong in a year?

David and I got heavily involved in the 1992 presidential campaign. We wanted the governor of Arkansas, Bill Clinton, to be the next president because of his plans for health-care reform.

My husband took me to my first Democratic caucus. I found it interesting. Everyone rallied for their candidate. David stood in front of the room and gave a speech as to why he thought Governor Clinton was a good choice. I was impressed on the great job my husband did. I always knew he was very smart. That night, at the caucus, he was elected to represent our district at the state capital.

Suddenly, our campaigning had to come to an end. I started to fall a lot. I kept getting weaker and weaker as the days went by. I struggled to climb the stairs to our home. I struggled to hang up my clothes. I didn't know what was happening to me.

I was afraid to go to the doctor because my husband had just purchased my health insurance. We both worried that they wouldn't cover me because the insurance policy was less than a month old. We wanted to wait at least three months. However, after a month had passed, I could no longer drive myself to work. I needed to see a doctor.

I began to stumble on cracks in the sidewalk. Simple activities like rolling up a car window became a struggle. I grew weaker and weaker day by day and minute by minute. It was like my muscles were deteriorating before my very eyes. Suddenly, I could no longer drive my car. It was too difficult to turn the steering wheel.

Dear God! What's happening to me?

How on earth did my husband know this was going to happen to me? He had to have seen it coming because why on earth would he have known to get health-care insurance for me just in the nick of time?

David had just purchased Blue Cross/Blue Shield health-care coverage for me not even thirty days prior. Was my husband psychic?

We knew something was very wrong with me, yet we put off going to see the doctor. David and I felt that if we went to the doctor right away, my problem might be seen as a preexisting condition and wouldn't be covered. We couldn't afford to take that chance. We could lose our home! We wanted to wait at least a few months. However, as time ticked on, I kept getting weaker and weaker. After two weeks, we felt we shouldn't put it off any longer.

My husband took me to see a primary care physician. David had researched my symptoms and believed that I was suffering from a condition called multiple sclerosis. The doctor gave me a routine examination and then scheduled an appointment for me to see a neurologist that very same day. David and I took the elevator up two floors to her office.

Dr. Abdawa gave me the same routine exam as the previous doctor. She asked me if I had been out of the country recently. She then turned to my husband and asked him to leave the room so she could do a thorough examination. I felt the doctor was uncomfortable with David's bombardment of questions and comments. My husband was always very curious. He also seemed extremely nervous. David started questioning everything the doctor was doing.

When my husband was out of the room, the doctor seemed relieved. She then turned to me and said that my husband seemed very overbearing. She asked if there was anything I needed to tell her about our relationship.

I explained to the doctor that David and I were still newlyweds. We had been married less than a year. I told her that he was probably as scared as I was about what was happening. My husband likes to have the answers. Here, we have no answers. This is the first time I have seen him lost and confused.

The doctor said that she was concerned about his behavior because she had dealt with abusive spouses who were responsible for their wife's illness.

I couldn't believe what the doctor was saying. I assured her that wasn't the case here. I told her that David would never do anything to harm me. She replied by saying that she just wanted to cover all her bases in trying to get to the root of the problem.

I never saw my husband as domineering. I always appreciated how he spoke on my behalf. I was never outspoken. I tended to keep things to myself. David was the opposite.

When I first met David, I let him decide on how I should dress because I was never good at fashion. He was a man who knew what looked good on a female. He was my Mr. Higgins in *My Fair Lady*. I valued his opinions and instructions. I always admired the fact that David had spent his life growing up studying to become a priest. He could make me a much better me than anyone, I thought. How on earth could the doctor believe that my husband could be making me sick!

I told her that my husband and I had a good relationship and that he was nervous, which makes him very outspoken and confrontational. I apologized for his behavior.

The doctor then requested blood work.

I was in the examining room for what seemed like hours. She wanted to know everything about me, including my job. She asked if I smoked and how much alcohol I drank per day. I don't know why, but I lied about my alcohol intake. I worked at a bar and drank a lot to be sociable. She asked where I went to school and how far I went in my education. I told her I graduated from Southern Illinois University in Edwardsville and had a master's degree in mass communication. I also told her that after graduate school, I spent the summer at a Baptist seminary in Kansas City.

Dr. Abdawa asked both my husband and me when we first noticed the symptoms. I didn't lie about when I started noticing that I was getting weak. However, I left off the fact that I had a bad cough prior to the weakness. I didn't tell the doctor about the cough because I didn't think it relevant at first. Weeks before I started getting weak, I had been drinking bottles of cough syrup, trying to suppress a nagging cough. The cough was so bad at times that I would lose my voice.

This made me wonder if the doctor was right. Could my husband be responsible for what was happening to me? His chain-smoking could have caused my cough. Our home always smelled of smoke. David would leave a cigarette burning in one room and light up another cigarette in the next room. Our ceiling and walls were yellowed with tobacco stains.

The cough probably started before I had health insurance. I couldn't risk not being covered due to a preexisting condition, so I never told the doctor about the cough.

David asked the doctor if she thought I had multiple sclerosis. The doctor said there were no specific tests to determine if I had multiple sclerosis. She would have to first rule out other conditions with similar symptoms.

The neurologist had blood work drawn to check for specific biomarkers associated with MS. The results came back showing a high elevation of enzymes. My CPK count was 40,000. Normal is 50. When a muscle is damaged, CPK (creatine phosphokinase, which is an enzyme in the body that is found mainly in the heart, brain, and skeletal muscle) leaks into the bloodstream. I was admitted into the hospital to undergo more tests, which included an MRI, spinal tap, evoked potential tests (measures electrical activity in the brain in response to stimulation of sight, sound, or touch), and muscle and lung biopsies.

Within an hour after being admitted, a team of doctors came into my room. The doctors had me perform activities like raising my arms above my head, lifting my legs off the bed, and sticking out my tongue. Each doctor then listened to my heart. There were so many doctors looking after me. I knew it wouldn't be long before I was diagnosed, treated, and sent home.

The following day, I was diagnosed with having sarcoidosis—a disease identified by the growth of tiny collections of inflammatory cells called granulomas, which were found around my lungs and muscles. Based on information from WebMD and Mayo Clinic websites, the cause of the disease is unknown. Experts think that bacteria, viruses, or chemicals might trigger the disease.

It wasn't a neurological condition. Dr. Abdawa transferred me to a rheumatologist named Dr. Kleermen. I was prescribed 60 mg of prednisone and released from the hospital a week after I had been admitted.

The doctor assured my husband and me that the disease is rarely fatal. She said that in some people, the disease may result in the deterioration of the affected organ—in my case, my muscles.

That tiny little pill called prednisone, a corticosteroid (manmade steroid) used to decrease inflammation and suppress an overactive immune system, was going to make me better! I called it my miracle pill!

I left the hospital feeling better than when I arrived. I wasn't stumbling when I walked. I didn't have trouble hanging my clothes in the closet. I could raise my arms above my head. I seemed to have my full strength back. I had worried for nothing. I felt so bad for suspecting my husband of having something to do with my illness. I never told him or anyone about my suspicions. It just lingered in the back of my mind. I really felt bad about suspecting my husband. He was as much a victim of that terrible disease as I had been.

I saw myself as a terrible wife. I wasn't used to having a man as caring as David had been throughout my sickness. He never let go of my hand when I walked from the parking lot to the doctor's office. He never left me alone at home. David never stopped looking at me the way he did when we first met. His affection never waned. How could I have even thought such ugly thoughts about the one person (other than my mom and my daughter) I could depend on?

We had an appointment to see Dr. Kleermen a week after I had been released from the hospital. There, she took another blood test to see if my CPK count was back to normal. Unfortunately, it was still extremely high. The doctor increased my prednisone dosage to 70 mg per day.

Three days later, I started going to the bathroom a lot. My husband took my temperature, and it was 104 degrees. He took me to the emergency room, and I was admitted. I had contracted a bladder infection. I was given antibiotics through an IV. I was in the hospital for a couple of days. During my stay, I had another blood test, which showed that my CPK count still wasn't even close to normal.

Dr. Kleermen increased my prednisone to 100 mg per day. I asked the doctor if anyone had ever died from sarcoidosis. She replied that although no one had died from the illness, patients have died from the side effects associated with treating the illness. That statement bothered me.

David started gathering more information from different websites and journals, including AFP (American Family Physician), about the drug I was taking. His research led to many disturbing findings.

Prednisone is an intermediate-acting corticosteroid first used in clinical practice in 1949 to treat rheumatoid arthritis before spanning to other practical uses, such as to treat blood disorders, breathing problems, severe allergies, skin diseases, cancer, eye problems, and immune system disorders. It is a corticosteroid that decreases your immune system's response to various diseases to reduce symptoms like swelling and allergic reactions.

My husband read that prednisone side effects can vary in severity and type depending on a person's overall health, age, and other medications they take. Women are more likely to experience prednisone side effects.

Prednisone, as an oral medication, which I was prescribed, can disrupt the balance of microorganisms in the mouth and sometimes cause side effects like thrush. It is also associated with sore throats, stomach pain, and digestive issues.

Common side effects highlighted on WebMD, Mayo Clinic, and journal websites include acne, abnormal bloating, blurred vision, headache, heartburn, scaling of the skin, trouble sleeping, nausea, sweating, muscle weakness, mood swings, elevated blood sugar levels, increased appetite, swelling, rash, and weight gain. Infrequent side effects include diabetes, Cushing's syndrome, puffy face from water retention, and irregular periods. Rare side effects include hallucinations, trouble breathing, seizures, enlarged liver, osteoporosis, fluid in the lungs, chronic heart failure, abnormal heart rhythm, and more!

People who have chronic inflammatory conditions such as rheumatoid arthritis, asthma, COPD, inflammatory bowel disease, or osteoarthritis are more likely to receive prednisone long-term—for several months or years. People who need to suppress the immune system for a long period of time, such as after a transplant, may also receive prednisone long-term. Likewise, my doctor was trying to suppress my immune system from attacking my muscles—particularly my proximal muscles.

Up to 40 percent of people taking long-term prednisone experience bone loss that leads to a fracture, according to an article by Dr. Muhammad Yasir and colleagues in the US Library of Medicine. Most people lose bone mass within the first six to twelve months of therapy.

About 1.3 percent of psychosis cases occurred in patients taking 40 mg or lower, while 18.4 percent occurred in patients taking 80 mg daily. Patients with a history of mental health issues and females are at greater risk.

Mental health symptoms start within three to four days after starting therapy, but they can occur at any time. Some people have symptoms, including depression, after stopping therapy.

Here are some reviews from September and October 2007 taken from WebMD website:

> Anonymous female between age 19–24, on prednisone for 1 to 6 months for Crohn's disease: "Way too much weight gain, and it takes forever to taper off of it."
>
> Anonymous: "First of all, I took prednisone for an extended period for Crohn's disease. The symptoms I had were weight gain (approx. 25–30 lb.), round face, acne, and terrible mood swings. I hated every minute of being on this drug."
>
> Anonymous female between age 35–44, on prednisone for 1 to 6 months for vasculitis: "60 mg per day to help with treatment of Takayasu. Sleep is hard to come by, dizzy spells, hot flashes, and moon face."
>
> Anonymous mother of two between age 25–34, on prednisone for less than one month for disease in which body has immune response against itself: "This medicine makes me sweat constantly, increased hunger, swelling, and mood swings."
>
> Female between age 25–34 on prednisone for ten-plus years for disease in which body has immune response against itself: "I have been off and on prednisone for years, and it is the only time I have ever felt 'normal.' I have been on 40 mg a day for about three weeks now and can finally walk, *sleep* a whole entire night without pain, my severe debilitating headaches have disappeared, the arthritic pain in my hands and heels have improved tremendously. For me, the

only side effect is heartburn, but I can deal with that considering it has given me part of my life back! I do not know what I will do if they taper me back off of it…"

Female between 25–34 on prednisone for one to six months: "Every side effect possible! I got Cushing's syndrome, diabetes, humpback, sweating, weight gain, *severe* osteonecrosis. Horrible experience."

Anonymous on prednisone for rheumatoid arthritis: "I *hate* the way I feel on prednisone, weight gain, constant hunger, mood swings, screwing with my new marriage! Have to find alternative!"

David and I began to worry about my treatment with prednisone, although the doctors were sure it was the right prescription if I had any chance of regaining my strength and getting my CPK back to normal.

Yet that powerful little pill was causing more damage than good, we thought.

My husband started questioning the doctor's methods. He told the doctor that the side effects seemed as bad as—if not worse than—the actual illness. The doctor told my husband that prednisone is used to treat immune system disorders. My immune system was attacking my muscles. There were no answers as to why. The doctor tried to assure my husband that it was the only treatment that could help me. She also promised him that the side effects would vanish as soon as I was taken off the medication.

Dr. Kleermen told us that once she got my CPK count back between 150 and 50, she would take me off prednisone.

In the meantime, I couldn't stand to look at myself in the mirror. My face was swollen like an oversized cantaloupe, and my stomach had swollen to the size of a basketball. The rest of my body was getting smaller and smaller from severe muscle loss. I looked like one of the starving children in third-world countries. My skin darkened. I grew facial hair. A rash spread across my forehead. Every time I looked in the mirror, I cried at what was looking back at me. Prednisone had me deformed.

I didn't know how on earth my husband could stand to look at me. I felt like a monster. I even began to act like a monster. I just wanted to shut myself in a dark room and not be bothered. I didn't want anyone to see me like this. I didn't want visitors (including family) in my home. I was angry at what had happened to me. I blamed myself for leaving the seminary. I accused God of being angry with me and pouring out his wrath! My world was collapsing around me.

The hospital bills started to arrive in the mail every day. Not one had been paid by the insurance company. They all were unpaid due to the pending investigation. What was happening? What was being investigated? The fact that I got sick right after I purchased medical insurance looked suspicious. If the insurance company didn't pay the bills, we would lose our home.

I had more than my health to worry about. This was causing stress in our marriage. My husband was becoming aggressive toward me.

My doctor told David to keep me exercising to build on what little muscles I had left. Tests had revealed so much scarring on my muscle tissue that my doctor wasn't sure if I would ever regain any of the muscles I had lost. It was my proximal muscles that were being destroyed. I had lost a lot of muscle mass, which could not be recovered once it was gone.

David would have me exercising from the minute I woke up until the minute I went to bed. I would fall from fatigue. My falls were lethal because I had no strength to block them. My arms and hands were no help to me.

One day, I fell and broke several of my ribs. There was pain in every breath I took. It was pure agony. I felt as if I was being tortured. My husband would put me in compromising positions where I could easily fall and break my neck. Though it would have been a quick death, which would have probably been the best way to die, it would also appear as an accident. I wasn't ready to die. I was going to be a grandmother. I wanted a chance to see my first grandchild. I didn't want to die.

Every day, I feared falling. The fear was overwhelming. It was so overwhelming that I started to despise my husband. I believed that if I didn't get away from him, I would lose my life.

David and I started to argue a lot. I became very resistant to anything he asked me to do. I felt he had become an abusive husband. One day, my mom came to visit me, and I begged her to take me home to live with her. I cried so hard, there was no way she could say no that day.

My husband came to visit me at my mom's a couple of days later. I asked my mom not to let him in the house because I was afraid for my life. My mom went outside to speak with him. I could hear my husband asking my mom if she noticed that my behavior wasn't normal. I couldn't hear my mom's response. David told my mom that I had been acting strange ever since the doctor had increased my medication to 100 mg. He said I hadn't been myself.

I felt a lot better the moment I moved in with my mom. I felt safe. She didn't force me to do things that would bring harm to me. Before my husband left that day, he handed my mom a small stack of mail to give to me. They were all medical bills. I opened each one. Each bill hadn't been paid by the insurance company. They were piling up. Not only was I worried about my deteriorating health, I had a pile of medical bills to worry about.

That following night, I heard a shotgun go off just outside my window. I started screaming for my mom to help me. I told her my husband had come back to kill me. "He wants me dead," I screamed. "All his troubles will be over once I am out of the picture."

I cried for my mom to call the police. She needed to hurry. The gunshots started to get louder and louder. My husband was approaching the front porch. I screamed at the top of my lungs for help. I screamed and screamed and screamed, and suddenly, I blacked out!

CHAPTER 5

Mercy for the Dead

The first time my husband sang a Gregorian chant to me in Latin, I was brought to my knees. Although I didn't understand what was being said, the words transported me to a wondrous place unlike any on earth.

My body seemed to be floating in space, my mind captured in the melody. I listened attentively as if my fate depended on it. Was I in mourning for my soul?

Dies Irae—Gregorian chant hymn from the traditional Catholic Requiem Mass (Funeral Mass)

The sequence "Dies Irae" is from the traditional Catholic Funeral Mass, or Requiem Mass, of the Latin rite. It is also prayed sometimes in the Divine Office. It is a long prayer with a very simple prayer, allowing us to meditate on death and the judgment and calling us to amend our own lives as we pray for mercy for the dead.

This version is chanted by the Benedictine monks of Santo Domingo de Silos. Below is the text of the Latin with the English version (translated by William Josiah Irons in 1849) beside. The Latin text below is taken from the Requiem Mass in the 1962 *Roman Missal*. This translation, edited for more conformance to the official Latin, is approved by the Catholic Church for use as the Funeral Mass sequence in the liturgy of the Anglican ordinariate.

A DOSE OF MADNESS!

I.	Dies iræ, dies illa,	Day of wrath and doom impending!
	Solvet sæclum in favilla:	David's word with Sibyl's blending,
	Teste David cum Sibyll a	Heaven and earth in ashes ending!
II.	Quantus tremor est futurus,	Oh, what fear man's bosom rendeth,
	Quando Iudex est venturus,	When from heaven the Judge descendeth
	Cuncta stricte discussurus!	On whose sentence all dependeth.
III.	Tuba, mirum spargens sonum	Wondrous sound the trumpet flingeth;
	Per sepulchra regionum,	Through earth's sepulchres it ringeth;
	Coget omnes ante thronum.	All before the throne it bringeth.
IV.	Mors stupebit, et natura,	Death is struck, and nature quaking,
	Cum resurget creatura,	All creation is awaking,
	Iudicanti responsura.	To its Judge an answer making.
V.	Liber scriptus proferetur,	Lo, the book, exactly worded,
	In quo totum continetur,	Wherein all hath been recorded,
	Unde mundus iudicetur	Thence shall judgement be awarded
VI.	Iudex ergo cum sedebit,	When the Judge his seat attaineth,
	Quidquid latet, apparebit:	And each hidden deed arraigneth,
	Nil inultum remanebit.	Nothing unavenged remaineth.
VII.	Quid sum miser tunc dicturus?	What shall I, frail man, be pleading?
	Quem patronum rogaturus,	Who for me be interceding,
	Cum vix iustus sit securus?	When the just are mercy needing?
VIII.	Rex tremendæ maiestatis,	King of Majesty tremendous,
	Qui salvandos salvas gratis,	Who dost free salvation send us,
	Salva me, fons pietatis.	Fount of pity, then befriend us!
IX.	Recordare, Iesu pie,	Think, kind Jesu!—my salvation
	Quod sum causa tuæ viæ:	Caused Thy wondrous Incarnation;
	Ne me perdas illa die.	Leave me not to reprobation.

X.	Quærens me, sedisti lassus:	Faint and weary, Thou hast sought me,
	Redemisti Crucem passus:	On the Cross of suffering bought me.
	Tantus labor non sit cassus.	Shall such grace be vainly brought me?
XI.	Iuste Iudex ultionis,	Righteous Judge, for sin's pollution
	Donum fac remissionis	Grant Thy gift of absolution,
	Ante diem rationis.	Ere the day of retribution.
XII.	Ingemisco, tamquam reus:	Guilty, now I pour my moaning,
	Culpa rubet vultus meus:	All my shame with anguish owning;
	Supplicanti parce, Deus.	Spare, O God, thy suppliant groaning!
XIII.	Qui Mariam absolvisti,	Through the sinful woman shriven,
	Et latronem exaudisti,	Through the dying thief forgiven,
	Mihi quoque spem dedisti.	Thou to me a hope hast given.
XIV.	Preces meæ non sunt dsignæ:	Worthless are my prayers and sighing,
	Sed tu bonus fac beniiregne,	Yet, good Lord, in grace complying,
	Ne perenni cremer igne.	Rescue me from fires undying.
XV.	Inter oves locum præsta,	With Thy sheep a place provide me,
	Et ab hædis me sequestra,	From the goats afar divide me,
	Statuens in parte dextra	To Thy right hand do Thou guide me.
XVI.	Confutatis maledictis,	When the wicked are confounded,
	Flammis acribus addictis,	Doomed to flames of woe unbounded,
	Voca me cum benedictis.	Call me with thy saints surrounded.
XVII.	Oro supplex et acclinis,	Low I kneel, with heart's submission,
	Cor contritum quasi cinis:	See, like ashes, my contrition,
	Gere curam mei finis.	Help me in my last condition.

A DOSE OF MADNESS!

XVIII. Lacrimosa dies illa,   Ah! that day of tears and mourning,
      Qua resurget ex favílla   From the dust of earth returning
      Iudicandus homo reus: Man for judgement must prepare him,
      Huic ergo parce, Deus: Spare, O God, in mercy spare him.

XIX.   Pie Iesu Domine,   Lord, all-pitying, Jesus blest,
      Dona eis requiem. Amen.   Grant them Thine eternal rest. Amen.

CHAPTER 6

My Second Wind

Have you ever heard an elderly person say to a younger person, "You are truly an old soul"?

I do believe in the afterlife. I believe that once we die, our souls find a new host. That when a person dies, there is a child being born somewhere in the world who will inherit their soul.

It was all happening as I lay in the hospital emergency room fighting for my life. Somewhere in the world, that same night, there was a pregnant woman with her husband in another hospital emergency room about to give birth. The woman had gone into labor. I was trying to turn her newborn into a stillborn as I fought to hold on to my old life.

It was a life I had grown accustomed to. I knew the people in this story. I was familiar with the scenery, and I had a past. Whereas a new life with new parents would be all new to me. It would be stepping into the unknown. The pain in the old life did not outweigh the fear of the new life. I would be starting all over in a story that hadn't been written. I didn't know the characters. And more importantly, a plot hadn't been developed yet.

It was my decision, and my decision alone, as to whether I would fight to keep my old life or start a new one with new characters. I still liked my old characters, especially my mother.

A disrupting voice came out of nowhere and drew my attention away.

"Please try to count backwards from one hundred."

I replied, "One hundred. Ninety-nine." And then I stopped due to an excruciating pounding in my head.

The following day was a repeat of yesterday. Nurses threw a towel over my head and pushed me in a wheelchair down the corridor to another secluded room in the hospital. They were desperately trying to keep me in hiding.

I had been begging for a weapon to defend myself from the stranger who wanted me dead. The nurses and doctors just ignored my request. They kept moving me from room to room. I never spent more than one day in a room. They were doing a good job in keeping me away from the evil father who wanted me dead so his child could be born.

There were moments when I had to hold my legs together tightly. I felt like I was trying to keep the pregnant lady's water from breaking. I didn't want her baby to be born. I hung on for dear life to the past I knew and the pain I had grown accustomed to.

Today, I was hurled into a part of the hospital wing that was still under construction. I was the only patient in that part of the hospital. I felt so vulnerable. I needed a weapon since there would be no one around to hear my cry.

I shouted out for a weapon but was ignored again.

Two nurses lifted me from the wheelchair and onto the bed. They then left the room. I noticed I wasn't alone.

There was a man sitting in the corner of the room. He looked familiar. He was writing in his notepad. The man stopped writing, looked up, and asked me if I knew what day it was.

I didn't.

The man then asked me to count backward from one hundred to one. I started counting. My head started pounding when I reached ninety-eight. I was unable to continue.

The man wrote in his notebook then stood up and left the room.

I pulled the covers over my head in fear of being alone in the room.

Minutes later, I heard someone enter my room. I peeped from beneath the covers to find a nurse standing over me. She was holding some pills for me to take. I told the nurse that if she would help me escape, I would go directly to the bank and get her a thousand dollars. I told her that I would get my bankbook as soon as my mom came to visit so I could show her how much money I had. I told her I would give her my bank card to make the withdrawal. All she had to do was take me to the airport.

The nurse looked at me attentively. Once I finished explaining to her how her good deed would save a life, she poured me a glass of water to take my medicine. She then said in a soft and gentle tone that she would do something a lot better to save my life. She said that she would pray for me. The nurse then left the room.

I couldn't believe how calm I became when the nurse left. It was as if the room had been filled with security. I didn't understand anything that had just happened. I just knew I wasn't afraid anymore. I began to wonder what was in that pill I had just taken.

I awoke the following day to find that same man sitting near the window in a corner of my room. Again, he was writing in his notebook.

This day wasn't a repeat of yesterday. I wasn't moved to another room.

The stranger in my room asked me if I knew where I was.

I told him that I was in the hospital.

He asked my name.

I told him my name.

He then introduced himself as Steve. He said he was a psychologist. He told me that I was brought to the hospital in an ambulance a couple of days ago. I had gone into psychosis due to the high dosage of prednisone. The doctors had to slowly decrease the dosage to bring me out of it. He asked me if I remembered telling everyone that my husband was trying to kill me. I said no. Steve told me that the staff had to put me on blackout to keep David from finding me. I couldn't believe what I was hearing. My head started to hurt bad.

Steve asked me to count backward from one hundred. I couldn't reach ninety-eight. My head felt as if it was going to explode.

The psychologist continued to visit my room every day. He always asked the same questions. He always asked me to count backward from one hundred. It took several days before I could count backward without experiencing the excruciating pain in my head.

Once I could make the count, Steve told me everything that had happened while I was out of it. He didn't leave anything out. He started from the beginning.

The nurses kept moving me from room to room every time someone had spotted my husband in the hospital. They did everything they could to keep David away from me. It was shocking to know that the doctors believed my husband to be a threat to me. I was told that several times during the week, the nurses would put a towel over my head and wheel me down the corridor at a fast pace. It had been a game to them to see how well they could keep me hidden. They even found it amusing that my doctor had trouble finding me at times. One day, I was taken to a part of the hospital wing that was under construction. I was the only patient in that part of the hospital for days.

Also, during that time, the doctors were slowly weaning me off the high dosage of prednisone. I came to the hospital on 100 mg of prednisone. I was now on 40 mg.

There was one thing the psychologist said that baffled me. He said that I was put on suicide watch the first week I was admitted. I don't know how on earth that could be true because I was doing everything to save my life. That just didn't make any sense.

I asked Steve if he believed in life after death. He talked about what he had read on reincarnation. He found that "reincarnation was a philosophical or religious concept that an aspect of a living being or human starts a new life in a different physical body or form after each death." The concept is known to be part of the samsara/ karma doctrine of cyclic existence. The psychologist said that samsara refers to the process in which souls (jivas) go through a sequence of human and animal forms. He continued by adding that the idea of reincarnation is found in many ancient cultures, and a belief in rebirth/ metempsychosis was held by historic Greek figures such as Pythagoras and Plato. It is also a common belief of various ancient and modern religions such as spiritism, theosophy, and Eckankar; and is found as well in many tribal societies around the world such as in Australia, East Asia, Siberia, and South America."

However, when I told the psychologist what I had experienced during psychosis, he seemed to have more of a scientific explanation to what was happening to me.

According to an article in *Time* titled "Beyond Death: The Science of the Afterlife," scientists have theorized since the 1980s that NDEs (near-death experiences) occur as a kind of physiological defense mechanism. In order to guard against damage during trauma, the brain releases protective chemicals that also happen to trigger intense hallucinations. This theory gained traction after scientists realized that virtually all the features of an NDE—a sense of moving through a tunnel, an out-of-body feeling, spiritual awe, visual hallucinations, intense memories—can be reproduced with a stiff dose of ketamine, a horse tranquilizer frequently used as a party drug.

The following day, when Steve entered my room, I told him that I needed a pastor, not a psychologist.

He asked me why I needed a pastor.

I told him it was because I didn't have a Bible. I now realized that all the time when I had been asking for a weapon, I should have been asking for a Bible.

A few days after I was no longer experiencing psychosis, I was moved to a physical rehab unit. There, I went through intensive physical rehabilitation in an effort to walk again. I had been bedridden ever since I was admitted. There was a lot of muscle atrophy. I went to physical therapy twice a day every day for two weeks. The first week, the therapist tried to stand me up from the wheelchair and have me take a step. I was too weak to stand.

The room where I took therapy was one huge and very bright room. There were all kinds of workout machines for building muscle strength. There were all kinds of gadgets for helping the disabled become independent. Yet nothing seemed to work for me.

There were parallel bars on one end of the room and stationary bicycles on the other end. I was too weak for either. Instead, I lay on one of the blue mats in the middle of the room and waited until my assigned therapist came to do range of motion with my limbs.

I would study the room while I lay there waiting. There were patients recovering from a stroke. They were walking around the room, building their stamina. There were patients recovering from hip replacement surgery, pedaling on the stationary bicycles. I watched every day as patients grew stronger and stronger. I wasn't one of those patients.

One day, I heard a nurse who was standing in the doorway looking in my direction. She pointed me out to the other nurses and said, "Look at that poor thing! She's as weak as an old dirty dishrag." That nurse's comment was like someone had taken an anchor and attached it to my neck. It weighed me down physically, emotionally, and mentally. Those words had become as destructive to my spirit as the prednisone had been to me. Where was my Samaritan?

Luke 10:25–37 (KJV) states the following:

> And, behold, a certain lawyer stood up, and tempted him, saying, Master, what shall I do to inherit eternal life?
>
> He said unto him, What is written in the law? How readest thou?
>
> And he answering said, *Thou shalt love the Lord thy God with all thy heart, and with all thy soul, and with all thy strength, and with all thy mind; and thy neighbour as thyself.*
>
> And he said unto him, Thou hast answered right: this do, and thou shalt live.
>
> But he, willing to justify himself, said unto Jesus, And who is my neighbour?
>
> And Jesus answering said, A certain man went down from Jerusalem to Jericho, and fell among thieves, which stripped him of his raiment, and wounded him, and departed, leaving him half dead.

> And by chance there came down a certain priest that way; and when he saw him, he passed by on the other side.
>
> And likewise a Levite, when he was at the place, came and looked on him, and passed by on the other side.
>
> But a certain Samaritan, as he journeyed, came where he was; and when he saw him, he had compassion on him.
>
> And went to him, and bound up his wounds, pouring in oil and wine, and set him on his own beast, and brought him to an inn, and took care of him.
>
> And on the morrow when he departed, he took out two pence, and gave them to the host, and said unto him, Take care of him; and whatsoever thou spendest more, when I come again, I will repay thee.
>
> Which now of these three, thinkest thou, was neighbour unto him that fell among the thieves?
>
> And he said, He that shewed mercy on him. Then said Jesus unto him, Go, and do thou like*wise* [italics mine].

It was then that I realized the doctors and nurses were avoiding me because they had given up on my chance of a full recovery. They were the ones crossing over to the other side as I lay on the mat. Their vision of my recovery was no longer the same as mine. They had lost all hope for me to recover. I only saw doom and gloom when they looked at me. I wasn't ready to give up. I was determined to not let their vision become my vision.

I didn't look forward to going to physical therapy. I didn't enjoy lying on the mat, watching all the other patients get better and better each day. It was as if the therapists and nurses had crossed over to the other side. No one seemed to be there to help me get better, to nurture me back to health. They had given up all hope.

I seemed to be the youngest person in therapy. There were a lot of patients in their seventies who could do things my thirty-three-year-old body couldn't. They made me feel as weak as I was. If there was any chance of me getting back on my feet, I felt it wouldn't be here. I needed my husband back in my life because I knew he wouldn't give up on me. Tears started to roll down my face.

An orderly wheeled me back into my room. There, I began to fight for my chance at a full recovery. I prayed to God like I never prayed before. I prayed for a way back. I prayed for strength to fight. I prayed for God to light my way. I prayed for forgiveness. I prayed for a second chance. I prayed for mercy. And I prayed for David back in my life. I prayed and prayed until I got my second wind!

The following morning, I forced a spoonful of eggs down. Each day, I forced myself to eat a little more than the day before. I knew I needed nourishment for strength.

The following week, my doctor entered the room to tell me she would be releasing me soon because she believed my condition had reached a plateau. The doctor asked me who would be taking me home. I told her that I wanted my husband to take me home. The doctor called my husband. That same day, David walked into my room with flowers. I was so happy to see him. I hadn't seen my husband in nearly a month. I hadn't smiled since then. That very day, when David walked into my room carrying flowers for me, it was like the sunrise I had longed for. David was my Samaritan!

David immediately opened the blinds to bring light into the room. He then dressed me and helped me to transfer from my bed to the wheelchair. He was going to take me outside so I could feel the sun on my face. I hadn't been outside since I was admitted to the hospital nearly a month ago. It would be nice to breathe in fresh air. It would be nice to hear something other than heart machines and nurses paging doctors on the intercom. My husband immediately broke hospital protocol and took me out to feel the wind across my face. It was so delightful!

Later that day, the doctor spoke with my husband. She invited him to attend physical therapy with me that week before I was released. The therapist wanted to show him how to do range-of-motion exercises with me at home. They also wanted him to order an electric wheelchair to take me home in.

David told them that he would prefer a manual one. The therapist and doctor insisted he order an electric wheelchair so I could have a little independence at home with the push of a button. David explained to them that we lived up four flights of stairs. There was no elevator. The electric wheelchair weighed close to a ton. He said that he wouldn't be able to take me on drives to the park. He wanted me to be able to leave the house occasionally. My husband didn't want me confined inside our home. He knew how much I enjoyed the outdoors.

The doctor told David he should have a stairlift built in the stairwell. David replied that we lived in a condo. He would have to get it approved by the condo association. He said he couldn't afford to purchase a stairlift even if the association would approve it. My husband went against doctor's orders and ordered a manual wheelchair.

The doctor and therapist both met with my husband to discuss my discharge. They told him that my condition had reached a plateau. I wasn't getting any better, but I wasn't getting any weaker either.

David did something that day that surprised both doctors and therapists. He stood me up in his arms, and I took a step. They were shocked. They asked him what kind of trick he just performed because what just happened was impossible. They told him that there was no way I could stand up because my muscle strength was a grade 2, which meant I couldn't stand up or do anything against gravity. They told David that what he did was impossible. The word *impossible* was never a part of my husband's or my vocabulary. We knew that with God, nothing was impossible!

When I looked into my husband's eyes, I could see a reflection of me when we first met. David still saw me full of energy and strength. He saw the woman he fell in love with. He hadn't given in to my present weakness like everyone else had. He saw me as he always had, and that reflection helped me to not lose sight of who I am and all that I am capable of!

Once David took me home from the hospital, we knew it was time to change doctors. The previous doctor had done all that she could. I wasn't ready to be at a plateau.

David called a rheumatologist named Dr. Moore. He had successfully treated conditions like mine. He and David had spoken on the phone for hours. David was sure we would have a fighting chance for a full recovery with this doctor.

Meanwhile, bills had piled up. The credit cards were maxed out. The disability check for $436 a month wasn't enough to cover the $600 mortgage.

My husband had to find a nurse to care for me so that he could look for work. But after he met a home health-care nurse who refused to ring the doorbell because it wasn't written in her instructions, David decided to get a job as a courier so he could take me to work with him on days my mother couldn't come to sit with me.

The courier business was a new experience for the both of us. It was exciting to learn to use the city maps and guidebooks in finding our way around Missouri. We twisted our way through newly built suburbs and discovered roads that led to old ghost towns. It was an adventure from the moment we got up each day. My husband—who was an overweight chain-smoker—would put me over his shoulders to carry me down four flights of stairs. I would always hold my breath until we reached the bottom.

It wasn't long after I had been released from the hospital that my husband had secured an appointment with Dr. Moore. There, I underwent much of the same tests as my previous doctor had given me. The results came back the same. The doctor told me the same as Dr. Kleermen had. The treatment was similar. The doctor put me back on prednisone.

I was hesitant when Dr. Moore wanted me to take 70 mg of prednisone per day. I asked him if he could find a different drug because I didn't want to go through those harsh side effects again. I told him that the side effects had been worse than the actual illness. I pleaded with the doctor to find another drug besides prednisone.

Dr. Moore said he understood my apprehension. He then promised that I would be on the drug for a short time. He assured me that I would be fully recovered and off prednisone by Christmas. That news perked me right up. Christmas was only three months away. The doctor prescribed 70 mg of prednisone per day along with 150 mg of Cytoxan, another immune suppressant. He then promised me that I would notice improvement immediately.

The only thing I noticed right off was the side effects of prednisone. My face and stomach puffed right up. My mood swings were back. My cravings for chocolate were back. My depressed state was back!

David took me back to the rheumatologist two weeks later. There was no improvement in my muscle strength. The doctor increased the prednisone dosage to 80 mg per day. He also added a third medication called methotrexate.

Christmas had come and gone and come again. My condition not only grew worse, I developed two more conditions. I was now being treated by three specialists: a rheumatologist, an endocrinologist, and a doctor of infectious diseases.

The rheumatologist was treating me for inflammation caused by sarcoidosis. His treatments included 80 mg of prednisone, 150 mg of Cytoxan, and 5 mg of methotrexate.

The endocrinologist was treating me for diabetes. I had developed symptoms due to the high dosage of prednisone. I had to be injected with insulin three times a day.

Lastly, the doctor of infectious diseases was treating me for tuberculosis. I had a TB skin test that showed a positive reading. Dr. Moore didn't believe the test was accurate, though he wanted me treated merely as a precaution.

The attention from all the specialists made me feel special at first. It was great to have so many professionals looking after me. Suddenly, my feet started to hurt. My husband and I believed it was a reaction to one of the many medications I was taking.

I went to see the rheumatologist about the pain in my feet. He said that I didn't have the pain when I was just taking his medication, so it couldn't be any of his treatments causing the pain. He told me I needed to tell the endocrinologist about the pain.

I told the endocrinologist about the pain in my feet. She said that none of her other patients were experiencing any pain like mine, so it couldn't be her treatment. The endocrinologist told me to tell the doctor of infectious diseases about the pain in my feet.

I told the doctor of infectious diseases about the pain in my feet. He said what the others had said. His treatments could not be causing the pain in my feet. He sent me back to the other doctors.

I developed a fever of 104 degrees while I was being treated by all the specialists.

David and I couldn't believe that not one of the doctors would take responsibility for the new problems I was experiencing. We became concerned about what would happen if something more serious surfaced. I felt as if I had been taken apart, and I needed to be put back together.

My husband and I immediately searched for a doctor in that same building who would be responsible for my entire well-being. We found a primary physician that same day after we left the office of the doctor of infectious diseases.

CHAPTER 7

A Bitter Pill to Swallow

I took myself off all the medication I was taking, including prednisone for the second time.

My husband and I decided I needed a doctor for all of me. I needed a doctor who would be responsible for all my well-being. We searched the directory for a primary care provider and found Dr. Bakanas. We chose her because her name was easy to pronounce.

Our first visit was different from any other of my visits to the doctor. I heard pounding footsteps coming toward the examining room where David and I waited. The door opened, and a tall woman entered. She was holding a thick file that contained all my medical records. I could tell she had done her homework.

She introduced herself to David and me with a firm handshake. The doctor then looked at me and apologized for all the medical procedures I had been bombarded with over the past year. She said she didn't expect to be greeted with such a warm and friendly smile after what doctors had put me through. She called me an amazingly good-spirited woman.

Dr. Bakanas not only showed empathy for what I had endured, she also acknowledged the pain my husband had endured as well. Unlike the previous doctors, she treated us as a couple who both needed healing. I immediately liked my new primary care doctor. She was already on the right track in bringing me comfort.

My husband, David, gave her a chart that showed all my medications, my dosage, my test results, my weight fluctuation, my mood swings, my side effects (including psychosis), and so forth. She studied the graph for quite a while. The doctor then looked up from the graph and complimented David for his impressive work. She even added that he might have just found the cure for his wife. Dr. Bakanas wanted to keep the graph and study it further before ordering any additional tests. I also gave the doctor a copy of the journal I kept. I told her that the information my husband used in constructing the graph came from entries in my journal.

When we decided to change doctors the first time, my husband bought me a journal so I could keep track of all my medical procedures. I tried to go back to day 1 from when I realized that something was wrong. Although I didn't know it at the time, this was the first major treatment in my successful recovery.

I was really impressed with Dr. Bakanas when she asked both my husband and me what were our expectations of her as our doctor. We told her that we needed her to be responsible for my entire well-being, including monitoring the treatments from the specialists. I added that I never wanted to take prednisone ever again. I truly believed that tiny bitter pill had done more harm than my illness. She responded by saying she couldn't make any promises to keep me off prednisone, but she could promise that it would be the last option after exhausting all other alternatives. She also said that she didn't want to put me through any painful procedures if she didn't have to, and that's why she wasn't going to prescribe any treatments until she looked at my husband's graph and my journal thoroughly. She then made an appointment for us to come back the following week.

I left the office that day feeling I had found the perfect doctor for me. Dr. Bakanas seemed to have my psychological, emotional, and physical well-being in mind. She was exactly what my husband and I needed.

We returned to her office the following week. The doctor had scheduled a few tests based on her findings. The test results supported her findings. Dr. Bakanas told me that prednisone was the right treatment the previous doctors had prescribed. However, it had been the dosage that had been mismanaged. I couldn't believe what I was hearing. The news was heart-wrenching. It was more than I could bear. I started to cry. No one knew what that damn drug had put me through. I tried to commit suicide when I was on that drug.

"That pill is evil," I cried. "Pure evil. Please find another way."

Approximately twenty-five years ahead are reviews on prednisone taken from the Everyday Health website:

> *07/2020 as anti-inflammatory.* "I started taking 20 mg of prednisone on Tuesday for pain and inflammation. I couldn't sleep, felt nauseous, lightheaded, dizzy, worn out, and completely like I'm going crazy! It's Friday and I didn't take one last night or today! I'm scared to death if I continue with my prescription, I will be full fledge panic attack, in the hospital, or dead! I don't recommend it at all!"
>
> *06/2020 for dermatitis.* "Was prescribed to take for six days. The first day to take six pills at 10 mg each. The second day to take five pills at 10 mg each. The third day to take four pills at 10 mg each, etc. Until the sixth day to take the last pill at 10 mg. Was prescribed short-term for poison ivy. By the fourth day, I was completely suicidal. My anxiety was through the roof. I had extreme panic and mania. Had I not had an Ativan on hand to take, I would have admitted myself to the psychiatric unit. Beware of this drug. It will rip away your sanity and mental health to the point where you think you've gone mad. I never want to feel that way again. It was terrifying."
>
> *05/2020 for asthma.* "I have a love-hate relationship with this drug. I normally burst into tears when I'm told I need to take it because the side effects are so bad, but it does help get me breathing when I'm really bad with my asthma.

The only way I counteract the rage that it brings is valium. Once I found out that valium helps force my body to rest and recover and settles my mind, it made me not so terrified. I only take the valium when I have to take the steroids. I also take a strong antacid as I had horrific esophageal spasm once (apparently, it's a similar pain to a heart attack). You'll most likely get fat and miserable on steroids, but at least you'll be able to breathe…"

Back to the mid-1990s, the doctor replied that prednisone had not been my enemy. She said it was the professionals in charge of administering it to me. She promised me that I wouldn't experience any of those previous harsh side effects under her supervision. The doctor pleaded with me to give her a chance to prove herself. Dr. Bakanas agreed that the minute I started experiencing any negative symptoms, she would take me off immediately. I was hesitant, but I wanted to give her a chance because I liked her and because she said it was the information from my husband's graph that led her to this decision.

Dr. Bakanas was the first doctor who seemed to know what to say to calm me. She called me courageous. She said that she saw something in me she'd never seen in any of her patients. She said I was a woman of "iron will." The doctor explained that a small dosage of prednisone was needed to manage the inflammation and stop the fevers. She said that my "iron will" had brought me so far and would carry me even further in life once the fever and inflammation were under control.

She started me back on 35 mg of prednisone. Unlike the doctors before, instead of increasing the dosage when it didn't seem to be affecting the illness, she lowered the dosage by 5 mg. She kept doing it until the blood-test results showed improvement. The doctor stopped lowering the dosage when she reached 20 mg. I stayed on 20 mg of prednisone for six months. A year later, I was on 5 mg of prednisone and starting to embrace my new normal.

Things gradually shaped up for me. Once the fevers and inflammation were under control, I started going to physical therapy three times a week. I never missed a session. Six months after going to Dr. Bakanas, I was able to stay at home alone. My husband put the couch up on four jack stands so I would be able to get off the couch without having to bend my knees.

Once a month, David would lower the four jack stands by a notch to see if I could still stand up. He did this hoping that, one day, the couch would be back on the floor. When he had the jack stands in the lowest notch, the couch was still about four inches off the floor.

My husband told our doctor about the jack stands. She suggested we purchase a lift-chair recliner. They were expensive. We asked the doctor if the insurance company would reimburse us for the lift-chair. She was afraid they would see it as a luxury instead of a necessity and not reimburse us. Yet she told me to write a letter to the insurance company and include the receipt, and she would give me a letter recommending the lift-chair recliner to me as a means of therapy.

I did write a letter explaining how the lift-chair recliner would benefit me more than a hospital bed. I was surprised that a couple of weeks after sending the letter, I received a check in the mail for the full amount of the lift-chair. That felt like the beginning of regaining my life after a long, drawn-out battle with this rare disease. When I told my doctor about the check from the insurance company, she was impressed.

Dr. Bakanas told me that she admired seeing my "iron will" in action. She said that thanks to me, she has witnessed the impossible become possible. She has seen success against all odds. She told me that she wished she could get a sample of my "iron will" and pass it out to the rest of her patients.

The doctor was also impressed when I started volunteering at the St. Louis Public Library three days a week. I told her it was my way of easing back into society after being away for what seemed like decades.

A DOSE OF MADNESS!

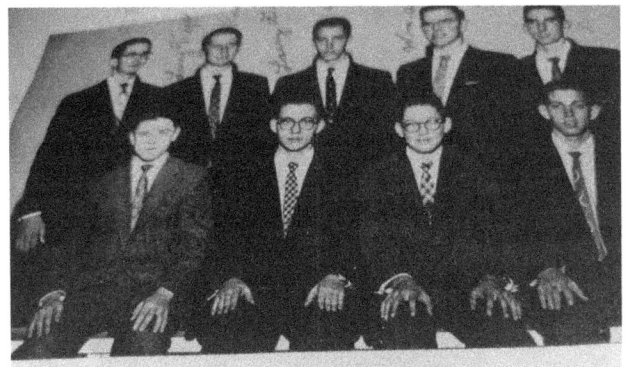

Top row (l. to r.) S. Courtois, R. Schoof, L. Guth, J. Behm, G. Gruber
Front row (l. to r.) L. Trapp, L. Green, W. Bogel, D. May.

The above picture was taken in 1958. It is a picture of the junior class at "The Cape" Preparatory Seminary of the Congregation of the Mission in Cape Girardeau, Missouri. David is in the front row and to the right.

The picture to the right was taken in 1959. David was a senior at "The Cape." David was on the yearbook staff, honor roll, baseball varsity, basketball varsity, handball varsity, and football varsity.

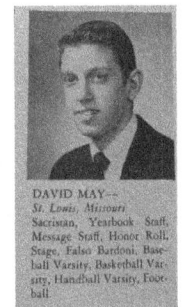

DAVID MAY—
St. Louis, Missouri
Sacristan, Yearbook Staff, Message Staff, Honor Roll, Stage, Falso Bardoni, Baseball Varsity, Basketball Varsity, Handball Varsity, Football

Although he was a member of the basketball varsity, it was his least favorite sport as an adult.

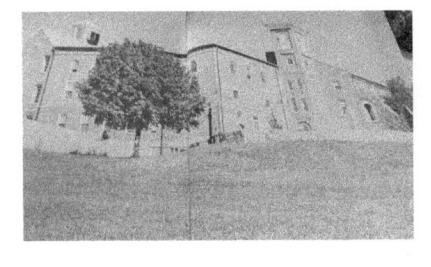

The picture to the left is outside "The Cape." The seminary trained candidates for the Catholic priesthood to serve in the Midwestern United States. The school was operated by the priests of the Congregation of the Mission (commonly referred to as the Vincentian Fathers) as a part of their mission since their founding in seventeenth-century France by St. Vincent de Paul.

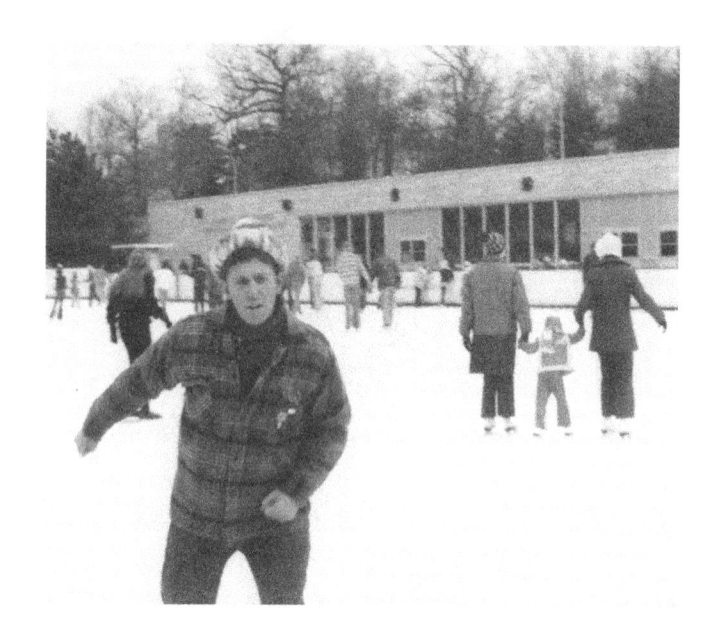

David's life after the seminary included ice skating (top picture) and visiting national parks (bottom picture).

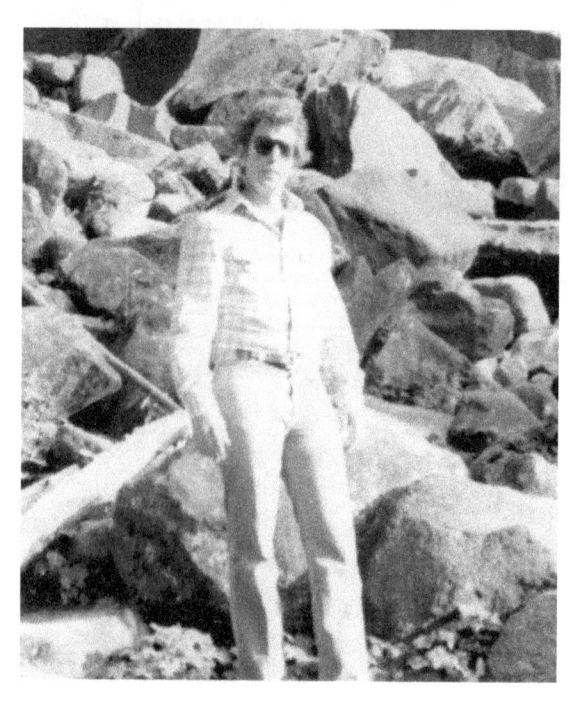

A DOSE OF MADNESS!

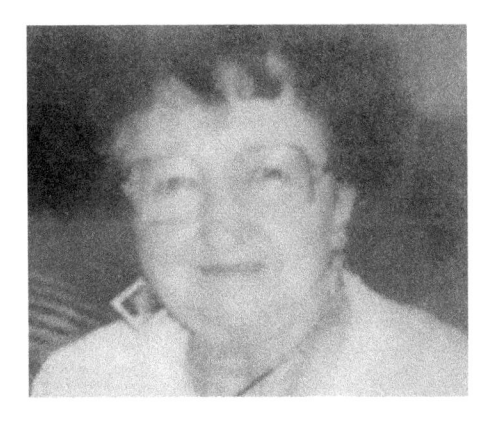

David's mother, Marie May (above photo), and David's father, Roy May (bottom photo), with his grandchildren, including David's two daughters, Leslie May and Stacey May (left side of bottom photo).

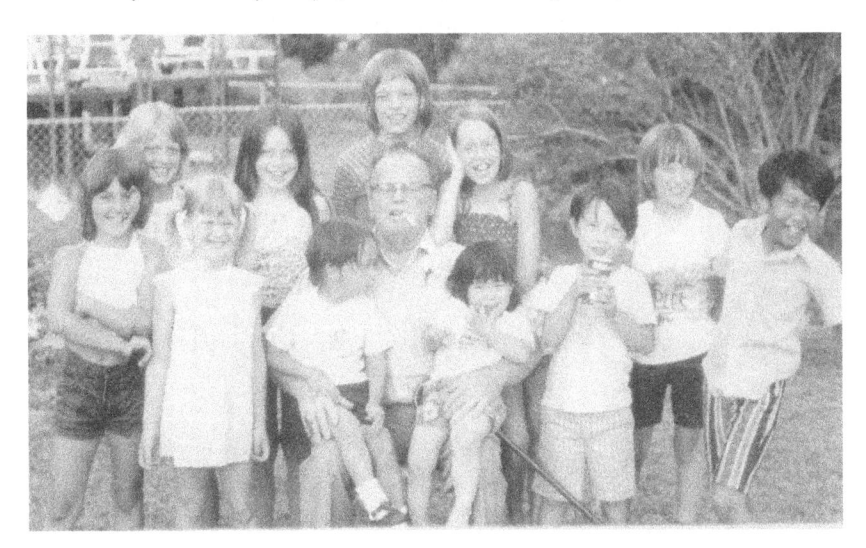

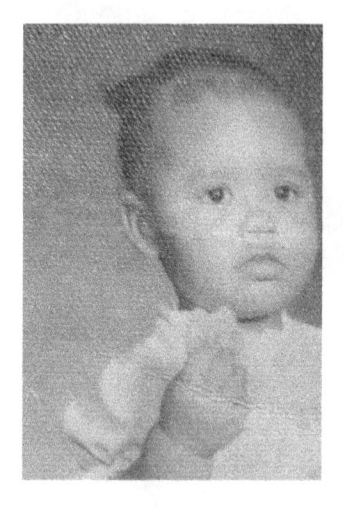

(Picture to the left) My daughter, Christie Eve Dale, was born December 24, 1976. Once she was born, I knew I had to get out into the world and make a living to provide for my daughter. The hardest thing I ever did in my life was leaving her to go to basic training.

I enlisted in the US Army in October 1977. Christie was ten months old when I left for basic training in Fort Jackson, South Carolina.

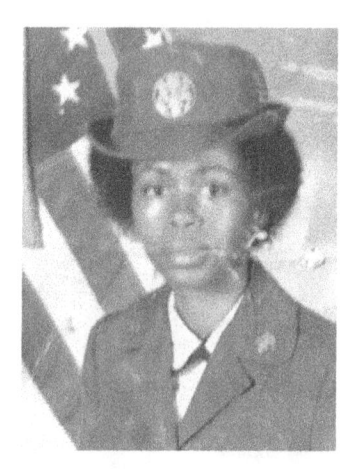

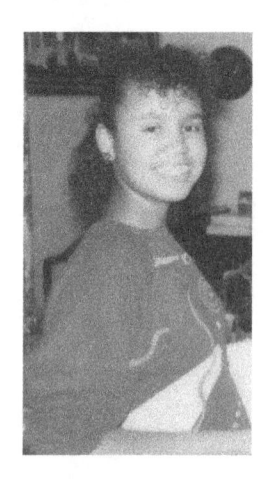

(Picture to the left) Christie Eve Dale is approximately twelve years old. I was in college. Unfortunately, I wasn't around much during this time of her life.

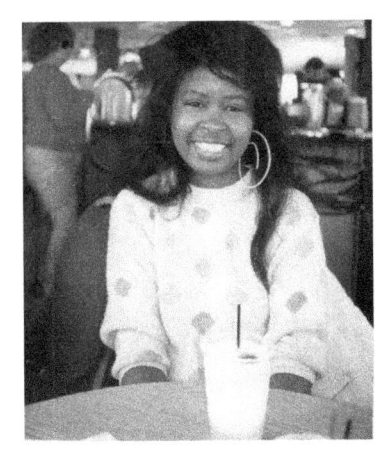

(Picture to left) David took a picture of me in Vegas, where I thought he was going to ask me to marry him.

(Picture to the right) David and I used to walk in Forest Park and dream about owning one of the mansions located across from the park.

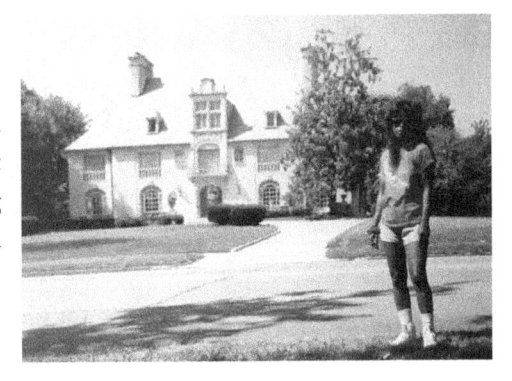

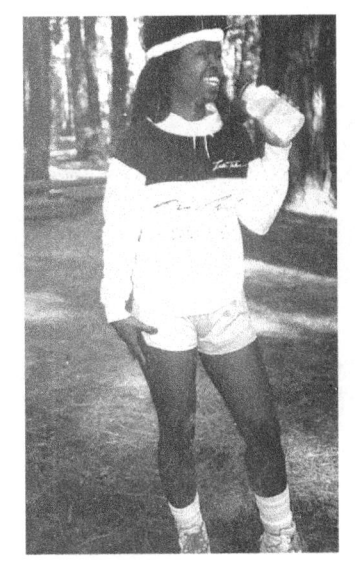

(Picture to the left) I was in my early thirties on a hike with David. While David and I were dating, he made me laugh a lot, no matter where I was or what I was doing.

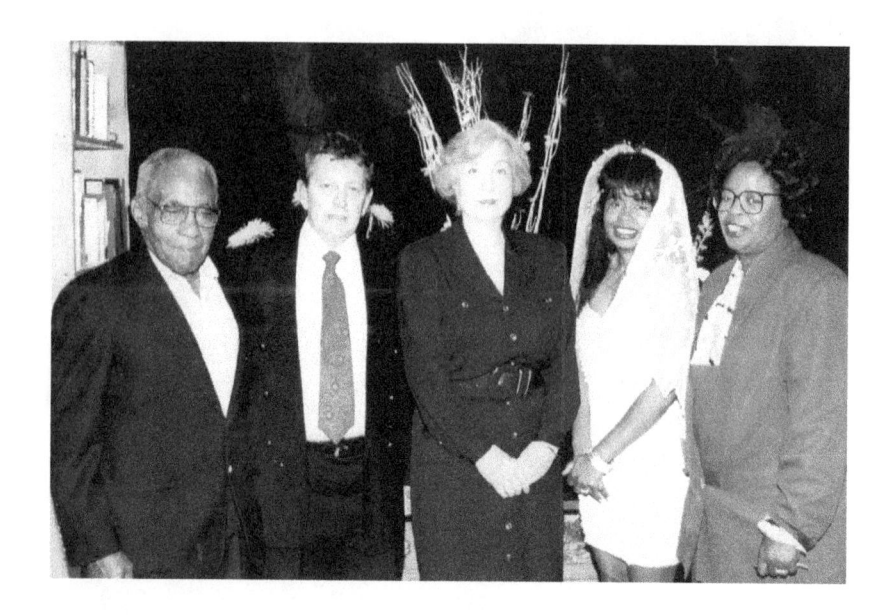

(Top picture) David and I married on October 6, 1991, in our home on Carroll Street in St. Louis, Missouri. (From left) My stepfather, James Kennebrew, David May, Rev. Phyllis Ferris (who performed the ceremony), myself, and my mother, Helen Kennebrew.

(Right picture) My husband, David, and I eating cake after the wedding ceremony!

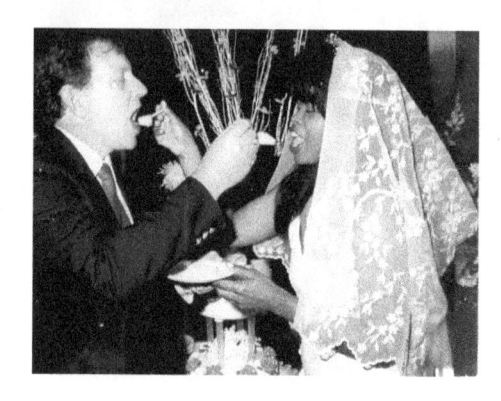

A DOSE OF MADNESS!

Right: During our honeymoon in Lake Tahoe before we drove to Yosemite National Park, David enjoyed lunch during a cruise in Lake Tahoe.

Centered bottom: David and I went horseback riding on a trail that overlooked Bill Cosby's home in Lake Tahoe.

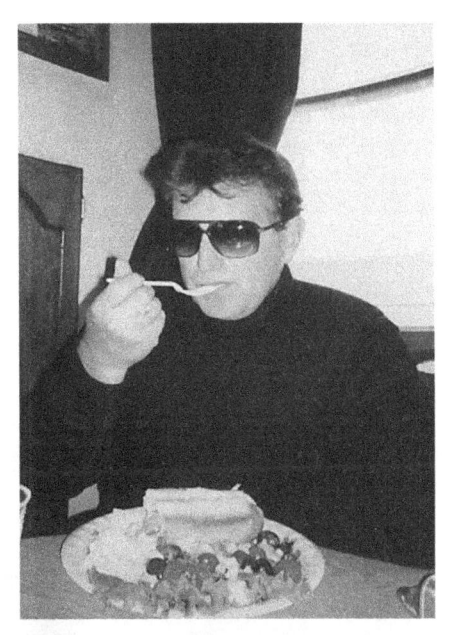

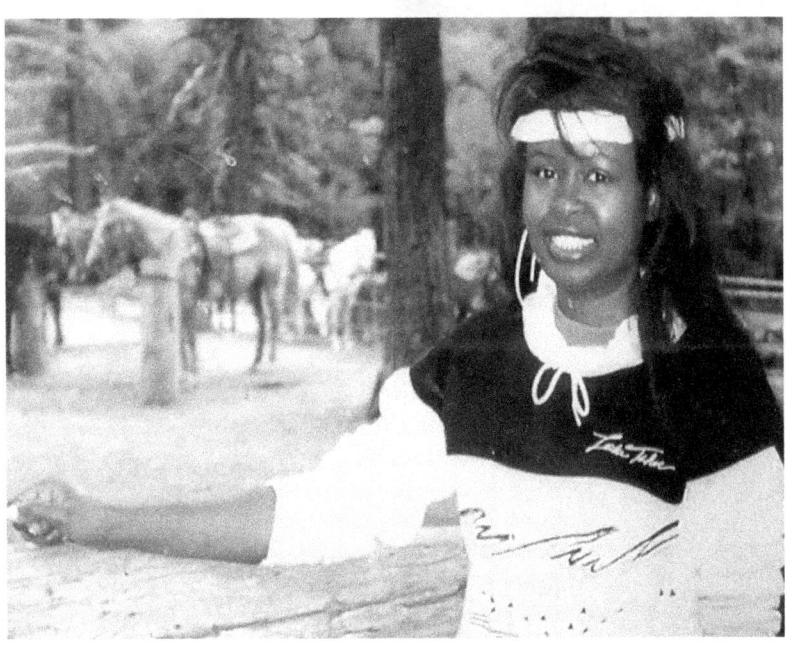

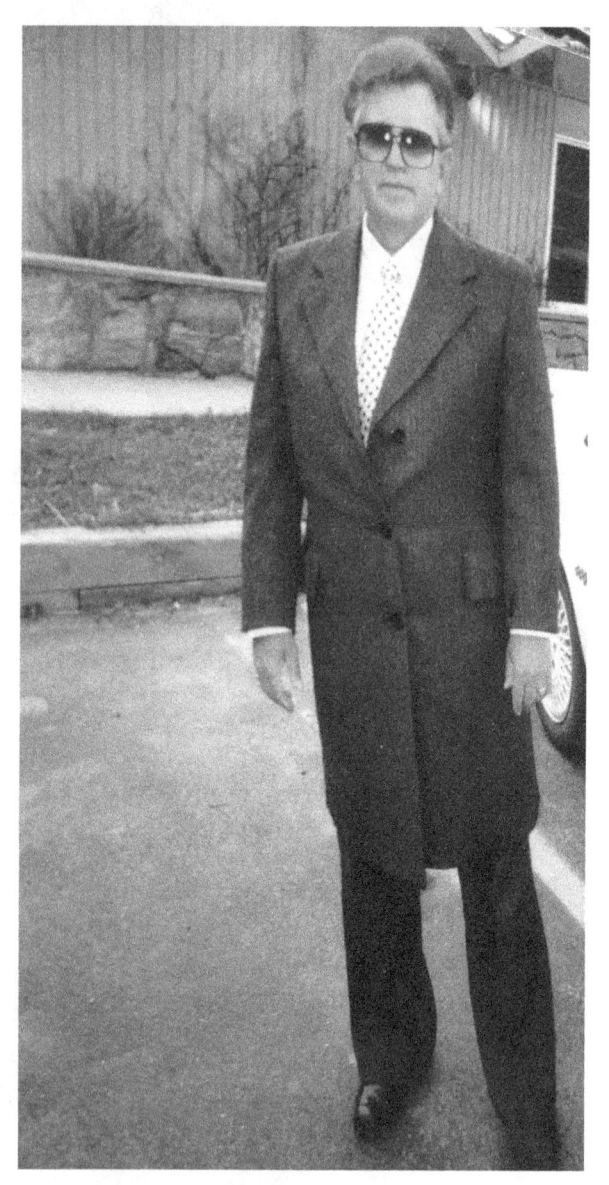

Above: David May in October 1991.

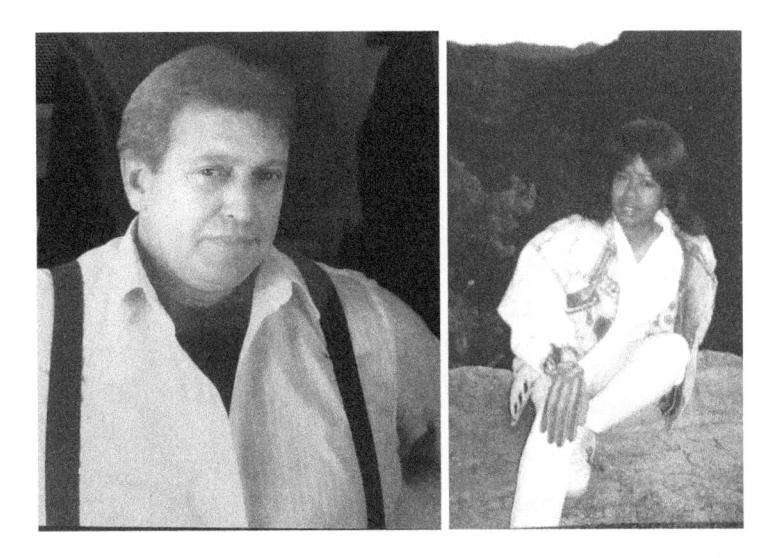

Top left: David May on honeymoon in Lake Tahoe.
Top right: Sheree May on honeymoon in Lake Tahoe.

Bottom: My daughter, Christie (centered), graduated from East St. Louis Senior High. My mother is to the left, and I am to the right. I still had my "moon face" due to the prednisone. I am still at the point where I need help getting out of a chair. I was able to walk before my daughter's graduation—not very good, but good enough to go without the wheelchair. God is oh so good!

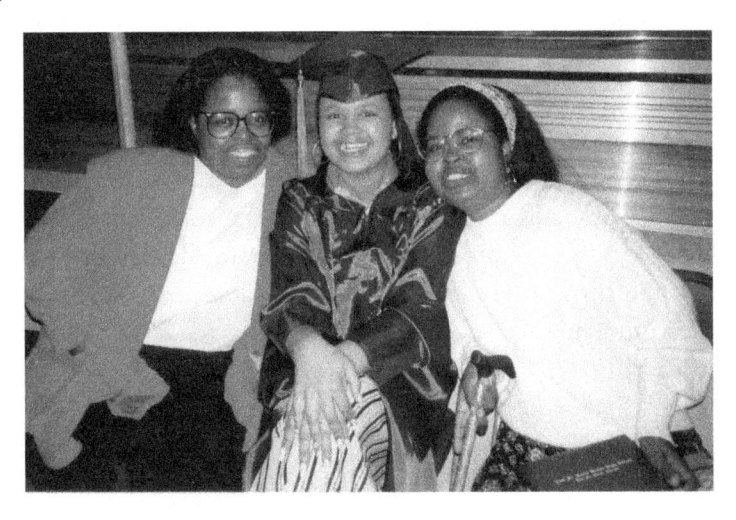

CHAPTER 8

On My Feet Again

I had been volunteering at the library for only a couple of months. I worked in the volunteer office that was tucked away in a corner on the third floor. My duties included answering the phone and calling on docents when a group from a school or organization scheduled a tour.

The manager of the volunteer department was John Soderberg. He interviewed me the day I came to volunteer. I liked being his assistant. John was a man after my own heart. Like my husband, he was working and caring for a sick wife. He would leave at lunchtime every day to go home and have lunch with his wife. One day, I gave him a package to take home and give to Mrs. Soderberg. It was a get-well card, a book titled *Chicken Soup for the Soul*, and snacks. I just wanted her to know that she was in my thoughts and prayers.

Volunteering at the library was good therapy. It was like walking into a fantasy world filled with paintings, stained glass windows, marbled statues, and more! The decor of the building was magnificent! People traveled from all over to come tour the library. I felt privileged to be surrounded by such beauty. Along with it came inspiration. I implemented a quarterly newsletter for library volunteers. John and I titled it *Volunteer Voice*.

It felt great to be able to put my education and skills to good use. John was impressed with my writing abilities. He said it took qualities not many people have, including himself. He told me I had a gift I should be proud of. I smiled and thanked him for the compliment. I never thought of it as anything special. I was happy to be able to contribute something beneficial to the volunteer program.

One of my goals for the program was to bring it from that secluded corner on the third floor into the limelight. I felt the newsletter would help me accomplish that. I interviewed the managers of each department of the library to see how volunteers could help them. I was taken aback to know that some of the staff looked on the volunteers as unreliable since they were not being paid to be there. I realized I had a bigger task ahead of me: to change the staff's opinion of volunteers. After all, I was a volunteer.

The docents had a more favorable reputation with the staff. They saw them as valuable since most were retired professionals like doctors, teachers, and entrepreneurs. Some of my favorite moments were spent sitting around the table and listening to the volunteers talk about their past experiences while stuffing envelopes for the marketing department.

The marketing department always had the most need for volunteers. They were always sending mail to the library Friends, inviting them to major events and book signings. I enjoyed volunteering at the library's special events. I got to meet famous people like Congresswoman Barbara Boxer, author Shelby Foote, and actor Danny Glover to name a few.

I remember how excited my husband became when I told him that Shelby Foote would be speaking at the library. He made sure he cleared his schedule to attend. My husband was a fan of the author. My daughter reacted the same when I told her Danny Glover was coming to the library. It was actually the first time I could get her to volunteer at an event.

Volunteering at the library had many perks such as meeting interesting people and celebrities, reading many great books, and being in an aesthetically pleasing environment. Yet my most priceless reward came from tutoring a seven-year-old girl named Ebony. I will never forget that feeling of accomplishment when she read a book to me and then told me about the story she had read. But that's not all. Her mother saw the good work I was doing for her youngest daughter, and she asked me if I would tutor her nine-year-old daughter as well.

My life once again had meaning. I had a purpose to wake up every day. I even started to dream again. My husband always called me a dreamer. I liked to dream big. My latest dream was to be able to work so that my husband could retire early. I wanted to make enough money to take my husband to Europe to visit the cathedrals. It was something he always talked about doing.

David had taken a job as a courier so that he could take me to work with him whenever he needed to. He worked a nine-to-five job delivering packages throughout St. Louis and the surrounding areas. I went to work with him when I couldn't stay at home alone. I watched my husband pick up large heavy boxes every day. It was backbreaking work. He delivered boxes in scorching hot weather and in knee-deep snow with temperatures below freezing. My husband never missed a day in ten years. More importantly, my husband never blamed me for having to work as a courier to support us throughout my sickness, even during the first six months when he had to carry me over his shoulders up and down four flights of stairs every day.

My husband was seventy pounds overweight and smoked two packs of cigarettes a day. He wasn't in the best of shape. Every day, when it was time for him to put me over his shoulders and carry me up or down those flights of stairs, I would hold my breath. I knew the best way I could show my appreciation for all he had done to support us was to be able to let him retire early and enjoy his life while I worked and supported the family. It would be a dream come true for me! However, I never wanted it to happen at the expense of another family.

One particular morning, I went to volunteer at the library as usual, but John wasn't there to let me into the office. It was the HR director who came and unlocked the door to the office. Something seemed off that day, but I couldn't quite put my finger on it. John never showed up to work that day.

After a week of no John, I asked the HR director if John was sick. He said he thought I knew that John's wife had passed away, and John was taking some time off. I told him that no one had told me the news. I was so sorry to hear that, and I took the news badly. I moped around the office several days afterward. I immediately mailed a sympathy card to John's address on file. I added a letter with the card expressing my deep sorrows and telling him to not worry about the office and that I would handle everything until he returned.

John had trained me well. I had pretty much run things in the office for years prior. I continued with the duties of manager of the volunteer department. However, several months had passed when I learned that John had moved to New York. He wasn't going to be returning to the library. The position of manager of the library's volunteer department had opened. I immediately applied for the position.

CHAPTER 9

The Promise

It's 7:00 a.m. I drag myself out of bed just as tired as I was when I had gone to bed the night before.

Every joint ached! Every muscle was sore!

I never realized how much work went into planning the annual library book sale event. There were days when I felt as if I had bit off more than I could chew.

I kept the volunteer department running when the director moved away. After his wife's death, he left the city to be near friends and relatives. There was no one to step in but his able volunteer. I had been volunteering at the library for over a year. I started the newsletter and increased the number of volunteers from eleven to seventy-five.

The director of human resources handed this project to me as a prerequisite to being hired permanently as the manager of the volunteer department. I eagerly took on the task in hopes of becoming a full-time employee so that I could receive the great benefits, including medical insurance for my husband and me. My husband still didn't have medical insurance. It would be the answer to my prayers.

I was eager to get the ball rolling, until I was taken to a building filled with boxes upon boxes upon boxes of books that needed to be unpacked, sorted, and repacked before the next annual book sale. The boxes were stacked from floor to ceiling. I couldn't believe my eyes. The next day, I got on the phone to recruit volunteers.

I remember when I brought my first volunteer into the room full of boxes. Her response was that there was no way she was going to spend her retirement doing manual labor. This included working in a dark and dusty room sorting books. She then walked out of the door never to be heard from again. That's when I realized that even my loyal volunteers had their limits.

Most of my volunteers were retired. I needed young physically fit volunteers for this particular task. I needed to look places I had never looked before to find them. This book sale wasn't going to happen if I couldn't get these boxes of books sorted. There were hundreds (maybe thousands) of boxes!

I started to pray every night for guidance. I needed able-bodied volunteers, and I needed them yesterday!

A few days later, a couple of young guys from the Church of Latter-day Saints walked into the office. My prayers had been answered! The young Saints started volunteering two days a week. They even brought four more young guys to assist. It was the best miracle I could have never imagined would happen to me. When the HR director walked into the building and saw six young volunteers busting through boxes of books, he couldn't believe his eyes. He looked at me in amazement. He called me a miracle worker. I had come to truly believe that I could do anything once I put prayer to it.

I don't think I gave God all the credit he deserved back then. I think I let my ego get in the way. I prayed every time I needed something, but I then took the credit when it happened. My relationship with God seemed to have been one-sided. My one-sided relationship would later suffer consequences, as always.

The day I received my first paycheck as an interim manager of the library volunteers, I felt on top of the world. It was nice to be able to hold down a job, although it was an interim position. David and I were going to take a vacation to New Mexico. He always wanted to go there to tour the oldest church in the country. My husband had an admiration for the architecture of old church buildings, especially Catholic churches.

I was excited to receive my first check. I was full of energy that day. I rolled up my sleeves and got dirty sorting through hundreds of books. I wanted to break my record of fifty boxes in one week. My volunteers had come and gone. I was still knee-deep in books. I was opening my seventieth box when I lost my balance and fell to the floor. I couldn't get up. I had never regained full strength in my proximal muscles because I had lost so much muscle mass during my illness. I use a cane for stability. I didn't have enough strength to get myself off the floor. Gravity was against me. I have very little chest muscles to use my arms to bear my weight or carry heavy boxes.

This was my new normal, which I had spent a lot of time finding ways to compensate for. I always feared falling since I had no way of getting up without the assistance of two people. I was alone. I prayed that no one came in and found me on the floor. The HR director would never hire me if he heard about this. I had to find a way to get up before a library employee found me. I was surround by boxes of books. I had to think and think fast.

I took three books out of the box that was on the floor beside me. I stacked the three one on top of the other. I then managed to pull myself on top of the three books. I then took a book and managed to slide it underneath my bottom. I was now sitting on top of four books. There was a small box full of books next to me. I lifted myself from the four hardbound books to the box. I was now sitting on a box of books. Now, if someone came in and found me sitting, I could pretend to be working by sorting through one of the boxes around me.

There was a stack of two boxes of books beside the wall where I was sitting on a box of books. The stack was too high for me to raise myself onto, so I took three books from another box and placed them under me until I was high enough to move from one box high to two boxes high. I was now high enough from the floor where I could get onto a chair. I then managed to pull a chair over to me without falling off the boxes of books.

It took over an hour from the time I fell until I was back in a standing position. I was amazed at how I was able to get off the floor. I had to rely on my brain muscle since I had very little physical muscles. It came through! I wanted to rejoice for my victory. I wished there had been an audience to witness my feat. I felt so proud of myself at that moment when I got back on my feet. I felt invincible, like nothing could keep me down, including the endless boxes of books!

It seemed like every time I cleared a section of boxes, someone would bring more boxes of books. There appeared to be no end to my work. Some days, I would say we won't be done in six months before the book sale event. Other days, when the six Saints came to volunteer, there was a glimpse of hope.

I would go home covered in dust. There, I would shower for what seemed like an hour. I would then go to bed exhausted. The only saving grace was the possibility of having a job when the book sale was over. I would be the manager of the library volunteer department instead of interim manager.

The director of HR was very nice to me. He told me that if I kept up the good work I was doing, it would all pay off. I believed him. I knew that some of the library staff saw me as a handicapped person who was a liability.

Eight months of sorting through tons and tons and tons of dusty old books were coming to an end. We were now three months from the library's annual book sale event. I never thought I would hear myself say it, but we would be ready!

Hundreds of tables were being set up in three large rooms. The labeled boxes of sorted books would be arranged on top of each table by category.

The event was being broadcast on local radio stations. There were also ads printed in local newspapers. The public had been informed. It was now time to recruit volunteers to staff the event. The library employees as well as volunteers signed up to be cashiers and floor clerks.

This was a three-day event. The first day would be Friday, which is called the preview night. There is a fee for entrance except for the library "Friends," the people who make a monetary donation to the library. The library's Friends are invited to all special events, including the annual book sale. Most of the library docents were also Friends.

The book sale event was now less than a week away. The hundreds of tables were covered with books. Several adjourning rooms stored the remaining boxes for the floor clerks to retrieve as vacant spaces became available on the tables. The rooms had boxes stacked from floor to ceiling. I had recruited over sixty volunteers to man the three-day event. This included cashiers, baggers, and floor clerks.

It was now only two days before the annual book sale event. The building where the event was to take place had been transformed in less than a year. I remember when the HR director walked me over to the building and opened the door to a disarranged room filled with boxes and boxes of books that had been donated. Some of the boxes had been stored in basements and had water-damaged books. The HR director handed me the keys and told me that if I could get this room ready in seven months, I might have a permanent position here at the library. He added that his supervisors weren't sure I could accomplish the task and that he wanted me to prove them wrong. At first, I thought this was some cruel joke. I kept waiting for someone to shake me out of this nightmare.

The day before the book sale event, I got a surprise visitor. I didn't see him enter the room. I was busy rearranging books on one of the many tables. I heard the door open but never looked up. Suddenly, a hand touched my shoulder. I looked up and saw that it was the previous manager of the volunteer department and my friend, John. He had traveled from New York to be here for support. I was so happy to see him. I immediately invited him to dinner that night so I could tell him everything I had been doing since he left.

Later that evening, my husband made dinner for my guest and me. John and I sat in the dining room while my husband cooked his favorite pasta. I asked John if I had forgotten anything for opening day tomorrow. John had overseen the library's annual book sale for the past several years. He was the expert in organizing library book sale events. He told me that everything looked great. I then noticed his demeanor changed when I told him what the HR director had promised if the event was successful. I added that I would have tough shoes to fill as manager of the volunteers, but I was grateful that I had learned from the best.

Preview night arrived. There was a long line of people waiting outside for the doors to open. There were reporters talking to the people in line, which mostly consisted of "Friends." These were people who made financial contributions regularly to the library. Inside, volunteers and library staff went to their stations to get ready to greet the crowd.

The doors opened at exactly 6:00 p.m. The crowd rushed into the room, grabbing boxes as they made their way to their preferred section. It was like a tornado had entered the room. I stood back and watched in awe. My first book sale event. Would it be a success?

I was so glad when the annual book sale was over. I gave a special party for the volunteers a week later. I wanted to thank them for a job well done. We toasted with champagne. Little did I know at the time that alcoholic beverages were prohibited on library premises. However, the party was not in the main library. It was in the building across the street, where the book sale had taken place. Yet it was part of the library.

I had invited the HR director. He made an announcement at the party that the book sale event had been a sellout. He thanked them for their hard work and made a toast. It wasn't until the day after the party that he told me no alcohol was permitted on library premises.

The Annual Library Booksale Event was a sellout success! It was over! It had been an exhausting task. I needed a break!

CHAPTER 10

When One Door Closes

My husband, David, and I took a vacation. We were driving to Santa Fe, New Mexico. I had never been there. David's brother Donald and his girlfriend Wanda were also going with us. It was a vacation well *deserved*. I was hoping that I would have news about the manager position before I left, but there was no word. Every time I asked the HR director about it, he would just say the department heads haven't gotten to it yet. He would then assure me that the position would be mine and to relax and stop worrying. He also said that by the time I returned from my vacation, the position would be waiting for me.

The morning of our trip, my husband packed the car, and we headed to pick up Donald and Wanda. My husband and his brother were very close. This was the first time we were all going on a vacation together. It was a fifteen-hour drive, which was plenty of time for lots of conversations. My husband, his brother, and Wanda lived in the same neighborhood as young adults. David had just returned from the seminary when he met Wanda. He was around seventeen years old.

Wanda and Donald were dating, but it never went further because she wasn't Catholic. She was a Lutheran, and Donald's mother played a major role in ending the relationship. She wanted her sons to marry Catholic women. It's amazing how Donald and Wanda parted and married within their religion to please their parents. They raised a family then, years later, after both went through a divorce, they found each other again.

During the drive from St. Louis to New Mexico, Wanda told me about the time she first met David. He had returned from the seminary. She said that she was sitting on their front porch when she heard a voice inside the house cursing like a sailor. She said she was shocked when Donald told her that David had just returned home from the seminary. Wanda said she couldn't believe that anyone with a mouth like David's could have spent years in the seminary, studying to become a priest.

David also had a temper. He was never physically abusive but very verbal. His mouth had caused many people to walk away from him or (if on the phone) hang up on him. My husband went to a psychologist for help a few years before we met. There, he said he discovered how he had been missing the one thing his mother never said to him: "You are a good boy!" Throughout his life, David struggled with the thought that he was never a "good" boy. He needed to hear those words from his mother. This had eaten away at him since childhood. He said that when he was studying at the seminary, he never wanted to go home during summer vacation. The priest at the seminary had to force him to go home for Christmas. David never believed that his mother missed him when he was away at school.

I sat in the car listening to Wanda's stories about my husband's younger days. I knew in my heart that my husband was a gentle soul. I truly believed God sent him to me because he knew I would get very ill. I needed someone like David to recover from such a sickness. His great discipline and huge appetite for answers to everything and anything were the tools needed for my recovery. David was a godsend!

I could never have said that about any other man I'd had a relationship with prior to meeting David.

We arrived in Santa Fe at 2:00 p.m. the following day. We checked into the Inn of the Governors, which was located just two blocks from the Santa Fe Plaza. David had selected the hotel because of the rave reviews for their breakfast. Wanda and I looked forward to their tea-and-sherry reception each afternoon. The rooms were small, but I always enjoyed a private and more intimate surrounding.

Once we settled into our rooms, we went to have lunch at La Fonda on the plaza. I ordered trout, and it was delicious. We discussed our plans for the rest of the day and the next.

David wanted to visit a couple of Catholic churches in Santa Fe. We started with the Cathedral Basilica of St. Francis of Assisi. My husband loved to study the architecture of Catholic churches. He wanted to learn about every detail that went into the construction of the church. He could spend hours in one church learning as much as he could. David was never patient at much, unless he was admiring the inside of a church, cathedral, or monastery. Prior to my illness, we had made plans to travel Europe just to visit the cathedrals. Europe was full of history. My husband could spend years there studying architecture and his second favorite subject, World War II.

The next day after breakfast, we visited San Miguel Chapel. It was the oldest church in the United States. San Miguel Chapel was said to be one of the best examples of preserved adobe architecture in Santa Fe. The structure consisted of sunbaked earthen bricks on stone. Inside, a simple all-adobe altar arrangement featured a two-tiered niche with the statue of Archangel Michael above and a tabernacle below. The statue of Archangel Michael was equipped with silver helmet and sword but missing his emblematic scales of justice. Oil paintings on canvas of saints surrounded the statue.

Later that same day, we visited the Loretto Chapel. It was known for its helix-shaped spiral staircase called the Miraculous Stair. It was said to have been the subject of legend, and the circumstances surrounding its construction and builder were claimed miraculous by the Sisters of Loretto. The chapel was known for its twenty-foot spiral staircase making two full turns, all without support from a newel or central pole. According to the story, several builders were sought but were not able to find a workable solution due to the confined space. In response, the nuns prayed for nine straight days to St. Joseph, the patron saint of carpenters. It was said that on the last day of the novena (which is a form of worship consisting of special prayers or services on nine successive days), a mysterious stranger appeared and offered to build the staircase. The stranger worked alone, using a few hand tools. He then disappeared without a trace once it was finished. He didn't collect pay, and not one of the Sisters ever got his name.

The staircase was an impressive work of carpentry, seeming to defy physics as it ascended twenty feet without any obvious means of support. David spent what seemed like hours studying the details in the construction of the spiral staircase. I spent more time admiring the details in the amazing story.

Our time in Santa Fe was way too short, yet I was eager to get back to St. Louis. There should be a job waiting for me there.

My first day back at the library turned into a quiet day. Not much was going on that day. There were no tours scheduled. I was getting ready to close the office and go home when the HR director walked in. He asked if I had a good vacation. I told him it was very nice. He then got right down to business. He said that the heads of the library departments had hired someone to take over as manager of the volunteer department. The news left me speechless. He continued by telling me that the new hire would start next week, and they wanted me to train her before I left. Words had evaded me. I just nodded in disbelief.

I went home that night feeling betrayed. I told my husband what had happened as he drove me home from work. I was crying hysterically. David tried to console me. The minute we were home, I went straight to my room and cried until I fell asleep from exhaustion.

I woke up the next day and went to work wanting answers. I made an appointment to see the director of the St. Louis Public Library. He had no answers for me. I left his office and went to speak with the HR director, who had promised me the job. He told me that there were five department managers at the meeting who voted on who they wanted to hire for the position. He said the vote was unanimous for the other person because she was better qualified. He told me that they had tried to hire her when John applied, but she was not available during that time.

I left the HR director's office and went back to my office. There, I called every volunteer and docent to let them know I would be leaving. They wanted to fight for me to stay on, but I asked them not to.

I told them that I didn't want to be somewhere I wasn't wanted. The unanimous vote told me how the staff at the library felt about me being there. I also wouldn't be able to handle being in the same building with the HR director every day after feeling betrayed by him.

Little did I know that my dream job was just around the corner at the time. I mean, literally around the corner. The following day after I was told I didn't get the job, I sent in a résumé to the *St. Louis Post-Dispatch* for the position of "Ad-visor." I always wanted to work for either a major newspaper or a popular magazine. I had applied at the *Post* twice before for the same position. This time, I listened to my brilliant husband, who told me to first call and interview the hiring manager. He told me I should find out what they look at on a résumé before calling the applicant for a face-to-face interview. The hiring manager only called applicants with at least a year of experience in sales.

As a result, I highlighted my year and a half of sales experience on my résumé. I was called the following day after I turned in my résumé! I was hired the following week! I assisted customers in placing their classified ads over the phone.

Two years later, I was promoted to Account Sales. My husband, David, and I paid off our debts. David was able to retire early and do what he always loved to do: take care of me! I wanted to give my husband the world when all he ever wanted was me!

On June 21, 2021, three and a half months prior to celebrating our thirtieth wedding anniversary, my husband, David, passed away.

APPENDIX A

Sheree's Journal Entries

Date: Fall 1991

Occupation: Self-employed

Symptoms: I have a nagging cough that comes and goes. I attribute my cough to being around heavy cigarette smokers.

Doctor: Haven't been to a doctor in over ten years.

Tests: n/a

Test Results: n/a

Diagnosis: n/a

Treatment: n/a

Diet: I am on a regular diet, although I probably eat one meal per day. I drink at least four shots of tequila per day to be sociable at work.

Weight: 117 lb.

Activity: David and I walk four miles in the park at least three times per week.

Prognosis: n/a

Comments: Overview of my life: Gave birth to a daughter on December 24, 1976. Enlisted into the army October 1977. Enrolled in college September 1981 as an undergraduate. Graduated from SIUE with a master's degree in August 1990. Attended summer courses at Central Baptist Seminary in 1990 to become a minister. I left the seminary the following fall. I got a job at a bar. There, I met a Catholic man who had studied to become a priest but left the seminary after years of study. A few years later, he married a Catholic woman and had children. He is now divorced. Although he was Catholic and I was Baptist, we had one thing in common that counted. David was the first man I met whom I could have a meaningful conversation with. I learned all about the Catholic religion, and he learned about the Baptist religion. David sung a Gregorian chant to me in Latin that penetrated through my heart. He read me his poems that made me fall for him even more. David and I met in September 1990. We married in October 1991.

A DOSE OF MADNESS!

Date: April 1992

Occupation: Self-employed

Symptoms: I cough so hard, I lose my voice sometimes. I am starting to lose my balance every now and then. My husband thinks I may have MS.

Doctor: I have not gone to the doctor because I just purchased health insurance.

Tests: n/a

Test Results: n/a

Diagnosis: n/a

Treatment: I am drinking bottles of over-the-counter cough syrup.

Diet: I haven't had much of an appetite due to the coughing.

Weight: 117 lb.

Activity: Working nights, which involves standing on my feet for hours at a time. Walking two miles in the park with husband several times a week.

Prognosis: n/a

Comments: My husband and I were walking around the neighborhood when I stumbled on a crack in the sidewalk and fell. I landed on my right knee. I was in great pain. David and I wanted to put off going to the doctor a little longer because we were afraid the insurance agent would claim my condition as preexisting since we had just purchased health insurance.

SHEREE MAY

Date: May 1992

Occupation: Quit job

Symptoms: Falling a lot. Having trouble climbing stairs, hanging up clothes, rolling down car window, driving, and the like.

Doctor: Although we wanted to wait a little longer, we couldn't put it off any longer. David took me to see the doctor on May 4, 1992.

Tests: Blood and urine test, X-rays, lung biopsy.

Test Results: Blood test revealed CPK count 40,000 (normal is between 50 and 100). X-ray revealed granulomas on lung.

Diagnosis: Sarcoidosis

Treatment: prednisone 60 mg

Diet: Regular

Weight: 115 lb.

Activity: No longer walking four miles in the park, no longer driving.

Prognosis: Full recovery

Comments: My first visit to the doctor. I was referred to a neurologist. My symptoms were similar to MS. The neurologist gave me a blood test, which revealed a high CPK. She admitted me into the hospital for additional tests. I was diagnosed with having sarcoidosis. The neurologist referred me to a rheumatologist before I was released from the hospital.

A DOSE OF MADNESS!

Date: June 1992

Occupation: Unemployed

Symptoms: Fever, muscle strength continues to decline

Doctor: Dr. Kleermen

Tests: Blood and urine tests, muscle biopsy, CAT scan, MRI, chest X-ray, ultrasound

Test Results: CPK count 11,000 and urinary infection

Diagnosis: Sarcoidosis and urinary infection

Treatment: Antibiotics through IV. Also increased prednisone dosage from 60 mg to 100 mg.

Diet: Regular

Weight: 102 lb.

Activity: None

Prognosis: Full recovery from infection in less than a week.

Comments: My blood test still revealed a high CPK count. I don't have much of an appetite. I am beginning to worry because insurance has not paid any of my medical bills.

SHEREE MAY

Date: July 1992

Occupation: Unemployed

Symptoms: Hallucinations

Doctor: Dr. Kleermen

Tests: Blood tests

Test Results: CPK count still high

Diagnosis: Sarcoidosis and psychosis due to high dosage of prednisone.

Treatment: Gradually lower prednisone dosage until patient comes out of psychosis.

Diet: Regular

Weight: 97 lb.

Activity: Bedridden

Prognosis: Unsure

Comments:

A DOSE OF MADNESS!

Date: August 1992

Occupation: Unemployed

Symptoms: Unable to walk, unable to turn over in bed, unable to fan a fly from face

Doctor: Dr. Kleermen

Tests: Blood and urine tests, chest X-ray, muscle biopsy, PAP smear, CAT scan, MRI

Test Results: CPK count 4,000. Still granulomas on lung.

Diagnosis: Sarcoidosis

Treatment: Took myself off prednisone after experiencing psychosis.

Diet: Regular

Weight: 97 lb.

Activity: Wheelchair bound. Therapist does range of motion to keep joints from locking.

Prognosis: Will never walk again

Comments: I hadn't seen my husband since the psychosis. I demanded doctors to contact my husband and allow him to come and take me home. I was released after being in the hospital nearly a month. Doctor and therapist requested that my husband order an electric wheelchair for me to go home in. David went against doctor's orders and ordered a manual wheelchair so that he would be able to take me outside for fresh air and sunshine every chance he could. He would carry me over his shoulders down four flights of stairs. He would not have been able to accomplish that with an electric wheelchair that weighed over a ton. Once I was home, I took myself off prednisone. I vowed to never take it again. I also decided it was time to change doctors because every time I looked into my doctor's face, I saw no hope for any chance of me getting back on my feet. I wasn't ready to lose hope like my doctors. My husband found a new doctor for me. He was a rheumatologist like my previous doctor. He had treated patients with similar diagnoses.

A DOSE OF MADNESS!

Date: September 1992

Occupation: Unemployed

Symptoms: Unchanged

Doctor: Dr. Moore

Tests: New doctor took me through all the previous tests and a TB skin test.

Test Results: CPK count 1,500 (lower number doesn't mean disease is lessening, it means I have lost so much muscle mass). TB skin test revealed positive.

Diagnosis: Sarcoidosis and tuberculosis

Treatment: prednisone 60 mg, Cytoxan 150 mg, methotrexate 5 mg

Diet: Regular

Weight: 100 lb.

Activity: Bedridden

Prognosis: Fully recovered by Christmas, which was only three months away!

Comments: This new doctor gave me hope. I agreed to take prednisone again, knowing that I would have to take it for only a few months. My husband had found a good doctor, and unlike the previous doctors, he had developed a good rapport with him.

SHEREE MAY

Date: April 1993

Occupation: Disabled

Symptoms: Developed a fever

Doctor: Dr. Moore, doctor of infectious diseases and endocrinologist

Tests: Blood and urine test, CAT scan, chest X-ray

Test Results: CPK count still high

Diagnosis: Sarcoidosis, diabetes, tuberculosis

Treatment: prednisone 10 mg + TB medication + insulin

Diet: Regular

Weight: 129 lb.

Activity: Physical therapy twice a week

Prognosis: Unsure

Comments: I have been seeing Dr. Moore for over six months. He promised I would be walking by Christmas, which has come and gone. Since then, I have been treated for diabetes and tuberculosis. I am seeing several specialists. I am taking several different medications. I have developed pain in my feet and a high-grade fever. Not one of the specialists will treat me for these new symptoms because they are blaming each other. I have decided to take myself off all medications, including prednisone. My husband and I are now searching for a doctor who will be responsible for my entire well-being.

A DOSE OF MADNESS!

Date: March 1994

Occupation: Disabled

Symptoms: Fever, pain in feet, night sweats, muscle weakness

Doctor: Dr. Bakanas (primary care physician)

Tests: Blood and urine tests, X-rays

Test Results: CPK count above normal

Diagnosis: Sarcoidosis, diabetes

Treatment: Took myself off prednisone for the second time.

Diet: Regular

Weight: 109 lb.

Activity: None

Prognosis: Unknown

Comments: My husband and I decided we needed a doctor who would be responsible for my entire well-being, including monitoring all the specialists' treatments. We picked Dr. Bakanas from the marquee in the same office as Dr. Moore and the other two specialists I had been seeing. We picked her because out of the three others, her name was easy to pronounce. At least, that is what I thought at first. Today, I truly believed it was God's choice for us. The moment Dr. Bakanas walked into the examining room where David and I waited, she seemed different than the previous doctors. I knew she had studied my medical records thoroughly because when she reached out to shake my hand, she complimented me on being able to have a warm greeting for her after all I had been through. She was the first sympathetic doctor I had met. During the interview, she looked at the graph my husband brought her. She then asked to keep it and study it further in order to find what tests she needed to schedule for me. The doctor said she wasn't going to put me through all the tests the previous doctors had. I felt she was already looking out for my emotional as well as physical well-being, which was a welcomed addition.

A DOSE OF MADNESS!

Date: April 1994

Occupation: Disabled

Symptoms: Fevers stopped

Doctor: Dr. Bakanas

Tests: Blood tests

Test Results: CPK count 300

Diagnosis: Sarcoidosis

Treatment: prednisone 20 mg

Diet: Regular

Weight: 113 lb.

Activity: Physical therapy twice a week

Prognosis: Dr. Bakanas said that I have shown an "iron will" that she believes will get me to a state of independence. She said that it was not possible to know how much of my muscle mass has been destroyed through the illness, but she knows that however much I have remaining, she truly believes I will build upon it to its fullest potential. She said that she sees me living a full and normal life to a ripe old age because I have shown the faith and determination that has already overcome so many obstacles.

Comments: During my third visit to Dr. Bakanas, she pointed to a spot on David's chart where I was on a low dosage of prednisone, and I had no fevers, my CPK count was lower than it had ever been, and I didn't need to take insulin. The doctor assured me that prednisone was the right treatment. She said it was the administering of the dosage that had been causing the complications. She said that the previous doctors started on a high dosage, and when my body wasn't responding to the medication, the doctors increased the dosage. Dr. Bakanas said she wanted to start me on a low dosage and continue to lower it until she could get it to its lowest dosage that will continue to keep the CPK count under control. After much hesitation to go back on prednisone, I reluctantly gave in and followed the doctor's orders. She promised that if I started to experience any of the negative side effects, she would take me off prednisone immediately.

A DOSE OF MADNESS!

Date: September 1994

Occupation: Library volunteer

Symptoms: None

Doctor: Dr. Bakanas

Tests: Blood test

Test Results: CPK count 200, which the doctor considered normal

Diagnosis: Sarcoidosis

Treatment: prednisone 5 mg

Diet: Regular

Weight: 122 lb.

Activity: Physical rehab twice a week

Prognosis: Sarcoidosis is in remission. No symptoms of diabetes or tuberculosis.

Comments: Dr. Bakanas congratulated David on the graph he presented to her. She was able to see what dosage of prednisone would be high enough to send the sarcoidosis into remission, yet low enough to not experience the harsh side effects. I walk with a cane for stability. I have not regained full strength in my proximal muscles. I cannot stand up from a low chair. I cannot climb stairs without a banister. I cannot drive an automobile. I started volunteering at the St. Louis Public Library in an effort to ease back into society and to challenge my new normal.

SHEREE MAY

Date: June 1995

Occupation: Interim library volunteer manager

Symptoms: None

Doctor: Dr. Bakanas

Tests: Blood test

Test Results: CPK count 200

Diagnosis: Sarcoidosis

Treatment: prednisone 5 mg

Diet: Regular

Weight: 125 lb.

Activity: Physical therapy twice a week

Prognosis: New normal

Comments: I have been put in charge of coordinating the annual library book sale. This is a big responsibility. I have been promised the permanent position of volunteer manager.

A DOSE OF MADNESS!

Date: June 2000

Occupation: Ad-visor

Symptoms: None

Doctor: Dr. Bakanas

Tests: Blood test

Test Results: CPK count 200

Diagnosis: Sarcoidosis in remission

Treatment: prednisone 5 mg

Diet: Atkins

Weight: 130 lb.

Activity: Walking one mile daily. Physical therapy twice per week.

Prognosis: Sarcoidosis in remission

Comments: I am working as an Ad-visor for the *St. Louis Post-Dispatch*. We have caught up on all our bills since I became ill. David has health insurance! We are now planning our third annual vacation!

APPENDIX B

Poems by David May (1978)

A Friend I Never Met

He had a lover's quarrel with the world
Could his have been the same as mine?
It hardly could be line for line.
Yet into his fray I seem to be hurled.

In "A Friend I Never Met," David was referring to his favorite poet, Robert Frost. The poem he wrote above refers to the poem titled "I Had a Lover's Quarrel with the World" by Robert Frost.

Being Without

I wrote and no one heard.
So I said it to myself.
Then laid it back on the shelf,
With the rest of the herd.

I poured into stemmed glass,
Watching the tiny bubbles rise.
Then wondered at their lack of size,
Hoping this time would pass.

There are people about,
All manner of noise and chatter.
Then it's not of any matter,
No relief for my doubt.

Even the walls are a reminder,
Full of their moaning and laughter.
Then I hoped for better after,
Knowing before had been kinder.

What's in a Question

Someone once asked me,
"What is a poet?"
"I don't know," said me.
"What's your thought on it?"

He looked with a smile.
Turned and walked away.
I wondered for a while,
Why he didn't stay.

Was he just the kind,
Who knew the answer
And wanted to find
One to say, "yes sir"?

Or was he the type,
Knowing no answer
His ignorance ripe,
None to discover?

I'll ask him someday.
Maybe he'll ask me.
Then what will I say?
Which sort will I be?
Neither one, I pray.
A third choice I see.

The Gold Coast—Another View

I came down out of the hills.
To the flat, where the seagulls
Gently float, screeching their cry,
Twixt the blues of sea and sky.

Sun, white sand, and crushed stone beach,
Is all that this place can teach.
Beautiful women abound.
Their shadows are full and round.

There are drugs to dull the mind,
Most of which are human kind.
Man-made streams run through the town.
Which keep the cost of sewers down.

There's a trickle in the glades.
Come winter, even that fades.
Snow has stayed far from this place,
Not allowed to slow the pace.
Smell of spring and fall can't come.
Barred is not the homeless bum.

The plants have become wary.
Sand makes uprooting easy.
The people aren't like the plant,
Have concern for roots, they can't.
No mountains reach for the moon.
Not so much as a sand dune.
Brown leaves never scratch the ground.
Children deprived of that sound.

SHEREE MAY

Oh yes, one can find a tree.
Far from the reach of the sea.
One tree doesn't make the woods,
Here man creates all the goods.

Friends Now and Then

There is one. I know well, not home tonight;
Out with a friend and maybe two or three.
A few drinks will oil their light chatter.
Then one will ask, "How's it with you and he?"
"Same, I'm afraid. Not sure he's right for me."

If only one of them who came her way,
Just one out there could have bothered to say,
"He's a good man who has done you no wrong.
"Your feel for him is right. This long to stay."
Said as a friend, "Doubt has become your song.
"From your same old tune, he is made to stray."

Those that doubt run when the sure come around.
The fearful seek the afraid and are found.
Some never tire hearing their words repeat,
Yet many are put to sleep by their sound.

None remarked, "A nicer one you couldn't meet,
"Raised in new dirt, plowed under your old ground."
I guess her friends in the nest would have frowned.

How is it that she who cares what they say,
Finds so many who let her have her way.

My Gate

I stood in the doorway watching
A small boy climbing on my fence.
He was having a high old time.
My strung wire, he was pretending
A castle wall and he a prince.

My eye followed a single strand
To its end, where men make their cross.
When I noticed my gate was ajar,
Why couldn't it close with its own hand?
Then it wouldn't need me for a boss.

Gate, you are a simple device,
Your hinges crucial to your life.
Yet need my hand to come alive,
When I'm through, you wait to entice,
Like a lover ache for a wife.

A complicated life it ain't.
What worry be there for a gate?
Skin diseases—your main complaint.
Rusting hinges and peeling paint,
Then there's me to mother your fate.

None would suggest a gate loving.
Yet does your wood ever feel joy?
Then with a smile, I remembered
You younger, in wide arc, swinging,
Holding the weight of this little boy.

A DOSE OF MADNESS!

I envy you, gate, knowing your route.
Letting in mine; keeping out theirs.
Swing always the same, then home again,
Knowing it's my choice in or out.
Whether horse, cow, just my neighbors.

Someday I'll shut for good this door.
My passing on may leave you sad.
Left alone, you'll have but one fate.
Both hinges broke, all slats battered.
So bad, a gate you'll be no more.
Mother no, then you'll need a dad.

I thought, "Who'll mourn for you, gate?"
Then, I guess, it's all for the best,
If my gate never knows the rest.

The Inevitable Stream

Dams were made to be broken.
The faces of those downstream,
With third eye always upstream.
Told me what I always knew,
In the end, the stream will win.

The dam and those below hold
A common fate—swept away.
As surely as the waves lay,
The castles of children low,
Your flow will scour its own mold.

Men may build it to the sky.
Your river will go under,
Or taking your time longer
Will build a ladder of sediment.
The dam, it will more than tie.

Some will beg, "Build me wider,"
But their middle cries, "I'm weak,
"Easy prey for any creek.
"More cement will do no good.
"Oh, dam, there is no answer."
Dams were made to be broken.
To nature, they're but a toy.
"Please, gracious waters, destroy
"The sculpture of man's defeat.
"In the end, the stream will win."

I Call Him Friend

He shook my hand.
Then talked of him.
And I of me.
Then did it again.
Our heads nodded.
"I know what you mean."

But were his eyes brown;
Would he know mine?

He bought a few rounds.
And so did I.
As men will do.
I told my tale.
Slapping his back.
Then he topped mine.
Slapping mine back.

We talked about
The game tonight.
Ant the one last night.
"Hey, I like you"
Just didn't fit in.

The game over.
My glass empty.
"Good seeing you."
"Yeah, me too."

We had laughed.
Was he my friend?
When we have cried,
I can be sure.

APPENDIX C

Poem by Robert Frost

Here is "I Had a Lover's Quarrel with the World" by Robert Frost. This was David's favorite poem, which he said defined him.

If this uncertain age in which we dwell
Were really as dark as I hear sages tell,
And I convinced that they were really sages,
I should not curse myself with it to hell,
But leaving not the chair I long have sat in,
I should betake me back ten thousand pages
To the world's undebatably dark ages,
And getting up my medieval Latin.
Seek converse common cause and brotherhood
(By all that's liberal—I should, I should)
With the poets who could calmly take the fate
Of being born at once too early and late,
And for those reasons kept from being great,
Yet singing but Dione in the wood
And *ver aspergit terram floribus*
They slowly led old Latin verse to rhyme
And to forget the ancient lengths of time,
And so began the modern world for us.

A DOSE OF MADNESS!

I'd say, O Master of the Palace School,
You were not Charles' nor anybody's fool:
Tell me as pedagogue to pedagogue,
You did not know that since King Charles did rule
You had no chance but to be minor, did you?
Your light was spent perhaps as in a fog
That at once kept you burning low and hid you.
The age may very well have been to blame
For your not having won to Virgil's fame.
But no one ever heard you make the claim.
You would not think you knew enough to judge
The age when full upon you. That's my point.
We have today and I could call their name
Who know exactly what is out of joint
To make their verse and their excuses lame.
They've tried to grasp with too much social fact
Too large a situation. You and I
Would be afraid if we should comprehend
And get outside of too much bad statistics
Our muscles never could again contract:
We never could recover human shape,
But must live lives out mentally agape,
Or die of philosophical distention.
That's how we feel—and we're no special mystics.

We can't appraise the time in which we act
But for the folly of it, let's pretend
We know enough to know it for adverse.
One more millennium's about to end.
Let's celebrate the event, my distant friend,
In publicly disputing which is worse,
The present age or your age. You and I
As schoolmen of repute should qualify
To wage a fine scholastical contention
As to whose age deserves the lower mark,
Or should I say the higher one, for dark.

I can just hear the way you make it go:
There's always something to be sorry for,
A sordid peace or an outrageous war.
Yes, yes, of course. We have the same convention.
The groundwork of all faith is human woe.
It was well worth preliminary mention.
There's nothing but injustice to be had,
No choice is left a poet, you might add,
But how to take the curse, tragic or comic.
It was well worth preliminary mention.
But let's go on to where our cases part,
If part they do. Let me propose a start.
(We're rivals in the badness of our case,
Remember, and must keep a solemn face.)
Space ails us moderns: we are sick with space.
Its contemplations makes us out as small
As a brief epidemic of microbes
That in a good glass may be seen to crawl
The patina of this the least of globes.
But have we there the advantage after all?
You were belittled into vilest worms
God hardly tolerated with his feet;
Which comes to the same thing in different terms.
We both are the belittled human race,
One as compared with God and one with space.
I had thought ours the more profound disgrace;
But doubtless this was only my conceit.
The cloister and the observatory saint
Take comfort in about the same complaint.
So science and religion really meet.

I can just about hear you call your Palace class:
Come learn the Latin *Eheu* for alas.
You may not want to use it and you may.
O paladins, the lesson for today
Is how to be unhappy yet polite.

A DOSE OF MADNESS!

And at the summons Roland, Olivier,
And every sheepish paladin and peer,
Being already more than proved in fight,
Sits down in school to try if he can write
Like Horace in the true Horatian vein,
Yet like a Christian disciplined to bend
His mind to thinking always of the end.
Memento mori and obey the Lord.
Art and religion love the somber chord.
Earth's a hard place in which to save the soul,
And could it be brought under state control,
So automatically we all were saved,
Its separateness from Heaven could be waived;
It might as well at once be kingdom-come.
(Perhaps it will be next millennium.)

But these are universals, not confined
To any one time, place, or human kind.
We're either nothing or a God's regret.
As ever when philosophers are met,
No matter where they stoutly mean to get,
Nor what particulars they reason from,
They are philosophers, and from old habit
They end up in the universal Whole
As unoriginal as any rabbit.

One age is like another for the soul.
I'm telling you. You haven't said a thing,
Unless I put it in your mouth to say.
I'm having the whole argument my way—
But in your favor—please to tell your King—
In having granted you all ages shine
With equal darkness, yours as dark as mine,
I'm liberal. You, you aristocrat,
Won't know exactly what I mean by that.
I mean so altruistically moral

SHEREE MAY

I never take my own side in a quarrel.
I'd lay my hand on his hand on his staff
Lean back and have my confidential laugh,
And tell him I had read his Epitaph.

It sent me to the graves the other day.
The only other there was far away
Across the landscape with a watering pot
At his devotions in a special plot.
And he was there resuscitating flowers
(Make no mistake about its being bones);
But I was only there to read the stones
To see what on the whole they had to say
About how long a man may think to live,
Which is becoming my concern of late.
And very wide the choice they seemed to give;
The ages ranging all the way from hours
To months and years and many, many years.
One man had lived one hundred years and eight.
But though we all may be inclined to wait
And follow some development of state,
Or see what comes of science and invention,
There is a limit to our time extension.
We all are doomed to broken-off careers,
And so's the nation, so's the total race.
The earth itself is liable to the fate
Of meaninglessly being broken off.
(And hence so many literary tears
At which my inclination is to scoff.)
I may have wept that any should have died
Or missed their chance, or not have been their best,
Or been their riches, fame, or love denied;
On me as much as any is the jest.
I take my incompleteness with the rest.
God bless himself can no one else be blessed.

A DOSE OF MADNESS!

I hold your doctrine of Memento Mori.
And were an epitaph to be my story
I'd have a short one ready for my own.
I would have written of me on my stone:
I had a lover's quarrel with the world.

ABOUT THE AUTHOR

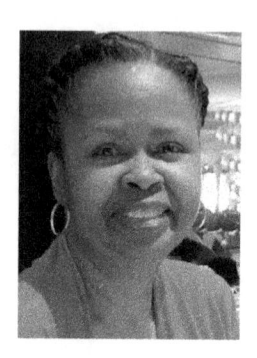

Sheree May has been a believer in a higher power ever since she was in grade school. Her military training, graduate studies, and work as a news editor has shaped her into a disciplined and detail-oriented writer. In acknowledgment of her exemplary work, she received a letter of recommendation from Dr. Constance Rockingham, dean of students at SIUE.

May is also the author of *Honor Thy Mother*, in which she talks about her journey as a caregiver to her mom who has Alzheimer's. May is currently widowed and lives in Florissant, Missouri.